Dr Clark is the first recipient of an award of distinction from the British Orthodontic Society for an outstanding contribution to the specialty of orthodontics. In 2008 he received an award from the International Functional Association for personal outstanding international service to functionalism and orthodontics. He has 55 years experience in orthodontic practice and is recognized as an innovator in orthodontics and dentofacial orthopaedics.

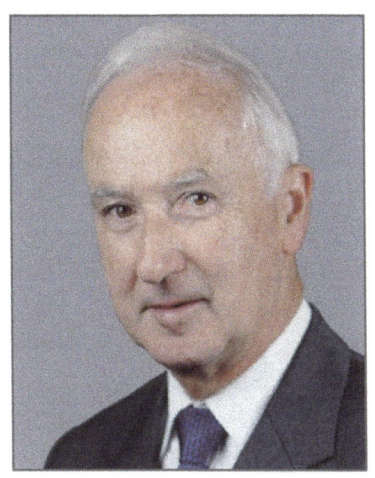

In 1977 he developed Twin Blocks and the technique is now used worldwide for functional mandibular advancement in treatment of mandibular retrusion.

In 2004 with Ortho Organisers he designed Invisible TransForce Orthodontics for interceptive treatment and arch development from mixed dentition to adult therapy.

Dr Clark has lectured worldwide over a period of 40 years in 55 countries. Courses on 'New Horizons in Orthodontics' offer practical advice on diagnosis, treatment planning and clinical management in fixed and functional appliance therapy.

A thesis "New Horizons in Orthodontics & Dentofacial Orthopaedics: Aspects of Twin Block Functional Therapy" at the University of Dundee gained the qualification "Doctor of Dental Science" after a lifetime of research in the field of orthodontics.

I0483281

Dedication

This book is dedicated to my patients. Without their good cooperation, I could not have achieved anything. I thank them for their permission to use their records in teaching orthodontics. It was a pleasure and a privilege to observe them complete their treatment and develop attractive and confident smiles.

William J. Clark

Published Text books:

W.J.Clark (1995) **– Twin Block Functional Therapy – Applications in Dentofacial Orthopaedics – 1st Edition** Mosby Wolf: English, Spanish and German Editions

W.J.Clark (2002) **– Twin Block Functional Therapy – Applications in Dentofacial Orthopaedics – 2nd Edition** Elsevier Science Ltd. English, Italian, Korean, Japanese and Russian Editions.

W.J.Clark (2014) **Twin Block Functional Therapy – Applications in Dentofacial Orthopaedics 3rd edition**. Jaypee Medical Publishers

W.J.Clark (2024) **Invisible Transforce Orthodontics (Available in digital format.)**

Dr William Clark 2023 - New Horizons in Life, Art & Poetry –Regency Publishers

For further information visit:

www.twinblocks.com   &   www.transforceorthodontics.com

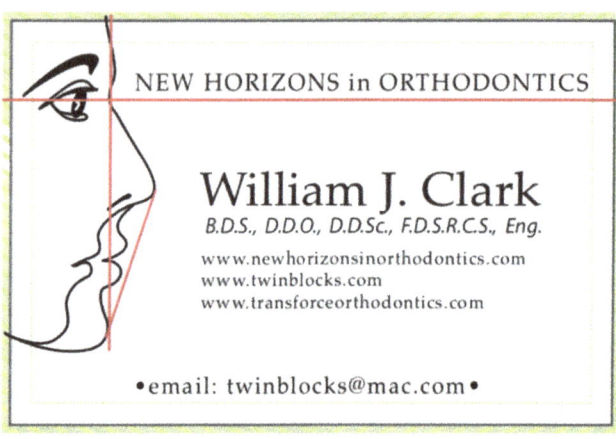

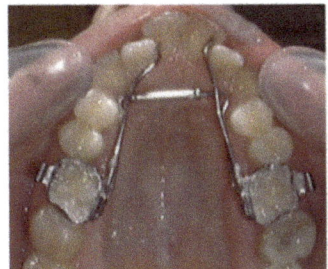

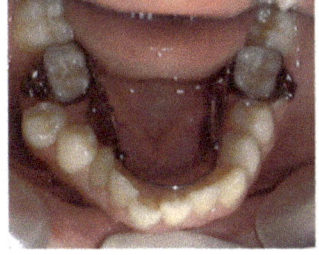

TransForce Orthodontics
Invisible TransForce Appliances

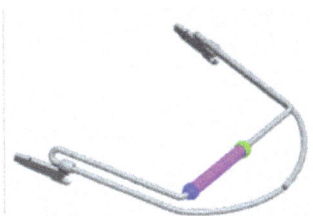

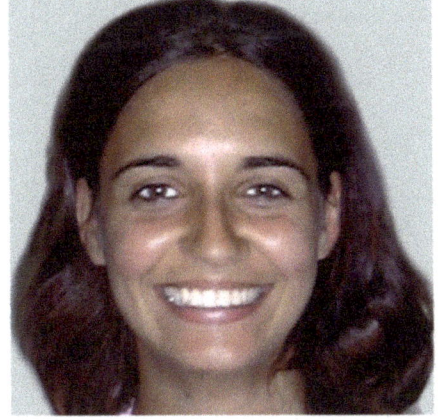

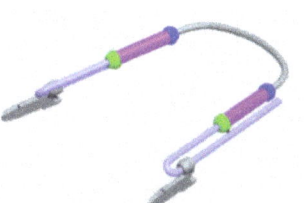

TransForm Your Orthodontics

William J Clark

B.D.S., D.D.O ., D.D.Sc.,F.D.S.R.C.S. Eng

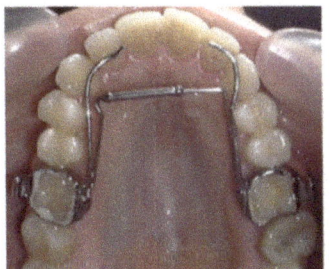

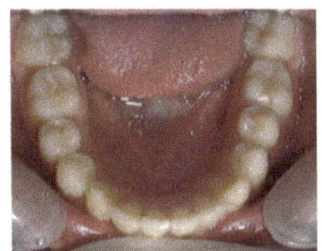

AUSTIN MACAULEY PUBLISHERS™

LONDON • CAMBRIDGE • NEW YORK • SHARJAH

A CIP catalogue record for this title is available from the British Library.

ISBN 9781528946131 (Paperback)
ISBN 9781528950046 (Hardback)
ISBN 9781528950053 (ePub e-book)

www.austinmacauley.co.uk

First Published 2024
Austin Macauley Publishers Ltd®
1 Canada Square
Canary Wharf
London
E14 5AA

Note
Medical knowledge is constantly changing. As new information becomes available, changes in treatment, procedures, equipment and the use of drugs and materials becomes necessary. The author and publishers have taken care to ensure that the information given in this text is acccurate and up to date. However, readers are strongly advised to confirm that the information, especially with regard to drugs and materials for intra-oral use complies with the latest legislation and standards of practice.

Introduction

The rate of technological change in contemporary society is accelerating, and orthodontics is not exempt from this process. In a highly developed specialty, it is only human to be comfortable with familiar concepts, as with familiar techniques, and to resist progress. The danger of complacency can apply equally in the academic or clinical environment. In challenging the status quo, the burden of proof rests with the innovator, and understandably there is a time lag between the development of new clinical techniques and their acceptance by the profession. It is encouraging to note that, with increasingly sophisticated methods of investigation, current research is providing consistent evidence to support the benefits of full-time appliances for functional therapy.

After a century of inconclusive evidence in the examination of orthopaedic techniques, the question of whether we can modify craniofacial growth by functional orthopaedic techniques remains to be resolved. A new paradigm for successful treatment presents a philosophical challenge to combine the benefits of orthodontic and orthopaedic techniques in the treatment of malocclusions which require a combination of dental and skeletal correction.

The question is fundamental to the organisation and delivery of treatment in the specialty of orthodontics. Past generations of orthodontists have based their treatment on the premise that we could not assist the mandible to grow beyond its genetic potential. Based on the early cephalometric studies of growth and development, this view was undoubtedly correct, until such time as new clinical and research techniques were developed to prove otherwise. Interpretation of the genetic paradigm is largely a matter of perspective. If the mandible is locked in a distal occlusion, it cannot necessarily fulfil its full genetic potential of forward growth, because it is trapped by an unfavourable functional environment. Unlocking the malocclusion may either help the mandible to grow or, by adjusting the direction of growth, allow the mandible to adopt a more forward position. New methods of research now confirm that full-time functional appliances are unquestionably more efficient in the correction of skeletal discrepancies than conventional fixed appliances.

Charting the course of orthodontics in the next century presents a challenge to consider alternatives to the techniques of the present day. While orthodontic practice is well equipped and organised to deliver comprehensive treatment in the permanent dentition, the same cannot be said for interceptive techniques, which do not yet receive the attention they deserve. Two-thirds of facial growth occurs by the age of 8 years. It is important to identify the benefits of early treatment to improve the form of the dental arches.

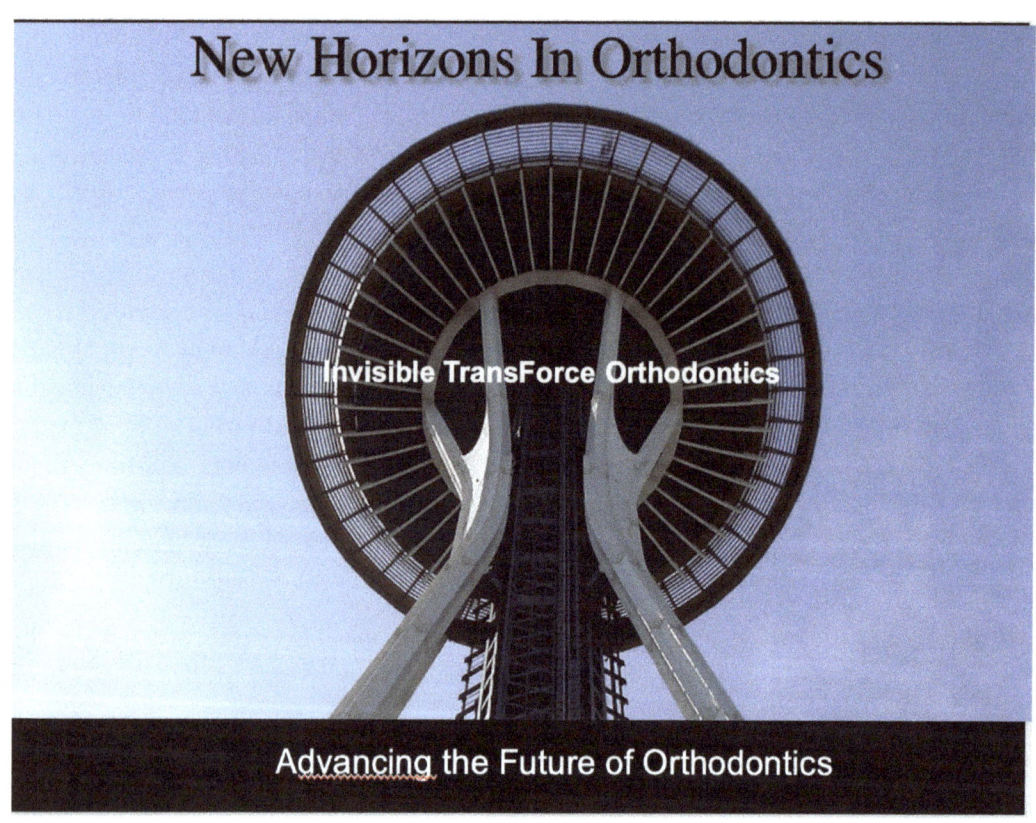

New Horizons In Orthodontics

Invisible TransForce Orthodontics

Advancing the Future of Orthodontics

Chapter 1

TransForce Orthodontics

Contemporary Treatment Protocol

The protocol for treatment in contemporary orthodontic practice is largely based on a labial approach using prescription bracket systems for correction of malocclusion in permanent dentition. Debate continues within the orthodontic specialty regarding the efficacy of early treatment, and the most advantageous time to commence orthodontic treatment. A lingual approach provides a valid alternative in the management of many malocclusions throughout the age range from early treatment in mixed dentition to effective adult treatment.

Three quarters of facial growth is complete by the age of eight. Primary dentition presents an important phase for treatment of major facial deformities including cleft palate. In the mixed dentition the maxillary and facial sutures are still responsive to adaptive bone growth within the sutures. Arch development techniques play an important part in the management of maxillary contraction by growth modification, whether in primary or mixed dentition. These techniques continue to be effective in the adolescent stage, provided light forces are applied to evoke a physiological response.

Maxillary Arch Development

Maxillary contraction is a common feature in all classes of malocclusion, and is frequently the primary aetiological factor, with secondary effects on the development of the mandible and the lower dental arch .

Consideration of the transverse dimension is important in the efficiency of orofacial functions. The airway may be restricted either in the antero-posterior or transverse dimensions.

A contracted maxilla is of particular significance, in view of its relationship to constriction of the nasal passages, with direct implications for the airway, and this has fundamental effects on general health. Patients with a restricted airway are subject to naso-pharyngeal infection and allergies, and their general health may be adversely affected. (Timms, 1968,1976)

Successful treatment of these conditions is firmly related to early interceptive treatment and is often associated with tooth-size/arch-size discrepancies. (McNamara & Brudon 1983). In many respects this is contrary to the present philosophy of a regimen for orthodontic practice based on treatment in the permanent dentition.

Based on histological studies, the prognosis for treatment of labial segment crowding is better in mixed dentition than in permanent dentition. Melsen (1972) carried out an investigation to determine the histological effect of rapid expansion of the mid-palatal suture in children of various ages. A true stimulation of sutural growth was found only in children who had not attained maximum pubertal growth.

In older individuals expansion resulted in numerous micro-fractures in the sutural region. The post-traumatic reaction around these fractures was of significance for the course of healing, preventing further growth in the suture from taking place.

Development of the maxilla to correct the archform is frequently the first step in treatment to unlock the malocclusion. The maxilla may be contracted antero-posteriorly or transversely, and often in both dimensions, when three-way expansion is indicated. Antero-posterior contraction is characterised by retroclined incisors, as commonly found in Class I bimaxillary retrusion, Class II division 2 and Class III malocclusion.

TRANSVERSE ARCH DEVELOPMENT

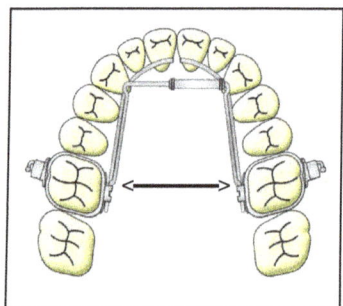

Transverse arch development is required to correct narrow arch form when arch width is restricted, either in the anterior or posterior segments.

Constricted arch width occurs in all classes of malocclusion and ideally should be treated in mixed dentition to promote normal function and encourage correct tongue positioning. A low tongue position is associated with a narrow palate and is often related to mouth breathing. Correcting arch width in early treatment offers the best prognosis for stability as the maxilla is more responsive to corrective forces before the permanent dentition is fully developed.

A narrow maxilla is a primary aetiological factor of upper anterior crowding, and may be responsible for secondary crowding in the lower dental arch. Maxillary constriction may predispose the patient to a distal occlusion and may restrict mandibular development in the sagittal or transverse dimensions.

On the basis of present concepts of dentofacial growth it is advisable to treat incisor crowding in the mixed dentition, when the incisors are erupting and the dental arches are amenable to transverse development. Parents frequently request treatment when they observe permanent incisors erupting in crowded positions.

Research has established that after the permanent canines have erupted the lower inter-canine width is an extremely stable dimension, and expansion in this region is unlikely to remain stable in the long term. The concept of interceptive treatment in mixed dentition is to expand the dental arches before the permanent teeth erupt to guide the premolars and canines to erupt in a wider arch form. Correcting tongue position may be a stabilizing factor following expansion of narrow arch form.

Significantly this treatment is carried out when the maxillary midline suture is more responsive to the forces of expansion, and low continuous forces may produce a more stable physiological response.

Frankel and Cetlin have previously demonstrated a stable increase in inter-canine width following treatment by a vestibular approach. The addition of a lip bumper may be an added advantage when combined with slow expansion from the lingual aspect.

Even in some Class II division I malocclusions the incisors must first be proclined or aligned to allow the mandible to be advanced fully into a class I relationship. In functional therapy arch development is often indicated as a preliminary to mandibular advancement in patients exhibiting crowding and irregularity in the dental arches.

The most natural method of arch development is by gentle pressure from the lingual aspect by the tongue. Lingual appliances for arch development simulate this natural process by applying gentle controlled forces to the lingual surfaces of the teeth, causing the teeth to migrate through the alveolar bone toward ideal arch form position. Lingual arch development is well established as a method of correcting arch form in interceptive treatment as a first phase of treatment prior to detailed orthodontic finishing.

There are significant advantages in directing corrective forces from the lingual aspect. The management of malocclusion in mixed dentition is improved by an efficient first phase appliance system. This approach can be used consistently to control a developing malocclusion at a stage when parents seek interceptive orthodontic treatment. Lingual appliances are used to relieve crowding, gain arch length, and correct arch form prior to functional therapy or fixed appliance finishing.

Arch development techniques are effective in the correction of all classes of malocclusion, and may be used at any stage of development from mixed dentition through permanent dentition with wide indications in adult treatment. Invisible lingual appliances are "patient friendly", and therefore acceptable to patients who might otherwise be reluctant to wear orthodontic appliances.

TRANSFORCE® LINGUAL APPLIANCES

The author worked with Ortho Organizers to develop TransForce Lingual Appliances as a new series of pre-adjusted fixed/removable appliances, which are designed to correct arch form for patients with contracted dental arches. Advanced technology was used to manufacture appliances with nickel titanium springs enclosed in a tubular compression unit. Transforce appliances control arch width and arch length by gentle spring-driven activation, combining ease of control, and a long range of action. Interceptive treatment with pre-activated lingual appliances offers new possibilities for arch development in combination with fixed appliances.

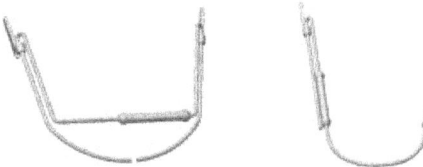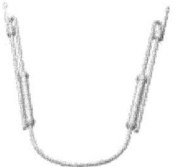

**Transverse & Sagittal TransForce Appliances
For Arch Development**

Spring driven forces, applied from the lingual aspect are used to activate a preformed lingual arch to extend archform by applying gentle pressure to the lingual surfaces of the teeth. The compression modules apply light continuous forces, similar to the forces applied by the tongue, to improve arch form from the lingual aspect. Several designs are available specifically to control archform in the sagittal and transverse dimensions.

Transforce® & Transforce 2® are registered trademark of Ortho Organizers

TRANSFORCE 2® TRANSVERSE EXPANDER

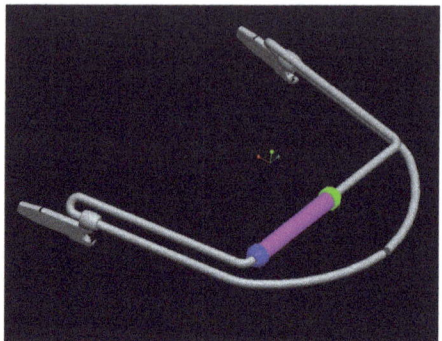

The Transverse Expander has an expansion module to increase the inter-canine width in upper or lower arches to accommodate crowding in the labial segments, or to correct arch width in contracted arches. This is an ideal replacement for the upper or lower Schwarz plate, by achieving a similar effect with a fixed/removable appliance, thus eliminating problems with the non-compliant patient. The Transverse expander is pre-activated to achieve the required amount of inter-canine expansion.

The appliance inserts in horizontal lingual sheaths on the molar bands and incorporates a gingival step mesial to the molar, placing the body wire close to gingival level. A recurved wire extends mesially from the molar sheath and may be used to align irregular anterior teeth from the lingual aspect. This facility is particularly useful when insufficient space exists to place brackets on lingually displaced teeth. The space is created first by transverse expansion before improving alignment prior to bonding brackets on the anterior teeth.

The expansion unit is positioned lingual to the incisors and is very effective in creating space in a crowded labial segment. However it is equally effective in expanding inter-molar width and widening the arch in the deciduous molar or premolar region. The body wire extends from the expansion module to be inserted in a horizontal lingual sheath on the molar band. Although the force delivered to the molar is reduced by the long lever arm, it is nevertheless an extremely efficient mechanism to increase molar width without tipping the molars, by delivering a low continuos force generated by the enclosed nickel titanium spring.

The Transverse Expander is provided in four sizes and the appropriate size can be selected for use in the upper or lower arch. The inter-canine width and inter-molar width is adjusted accordingly. The range of action of the Transverse appliance is 8 mm. The anterior transverse width of the appliance increases in 2 mm increments throughout the series. The mesio-distal length also increases by 2 mm to allow for variation in tooth width.

TransForce ®2 Transverse

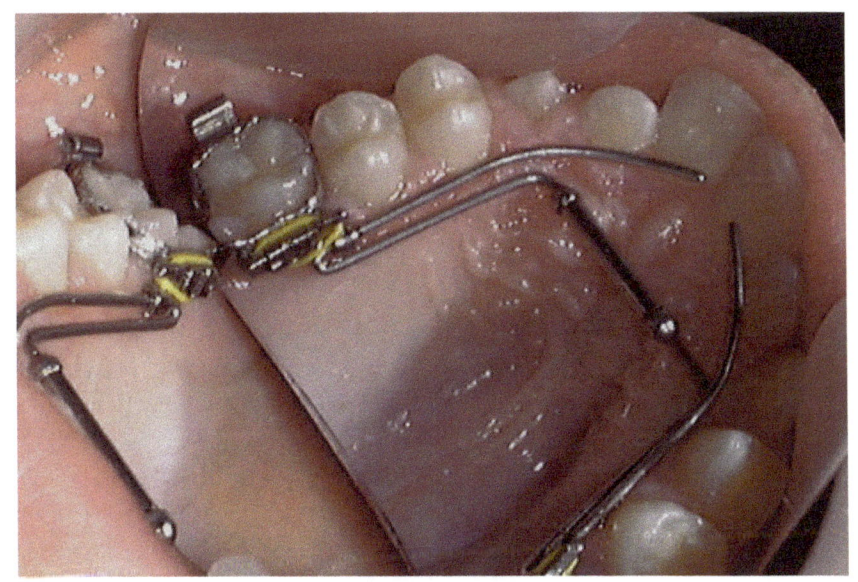

Aesthetic, Comfortable & Efficient

TransForce Transverse Expander

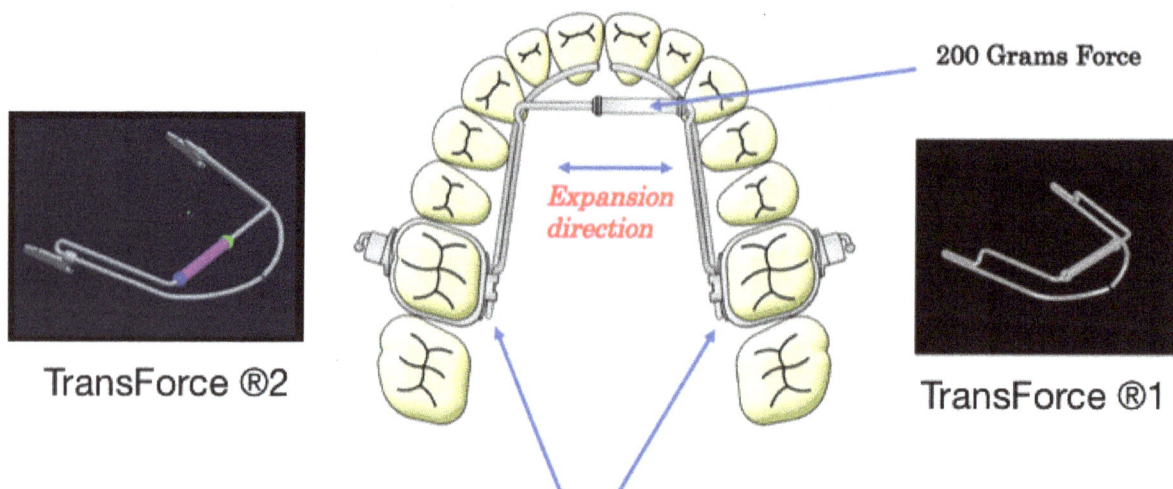

TransForce ®2

200 Grams Force

Expansion direction

TransForce ®1

Fits into Lingual Sheath

4 Sizes at 2 mm increments

The process of selecting the correct size of the Transverse Expander uses a similar clear template showing a scale model of the appliance in both compressed and fully extended forms. The template is laid over a study model to select the size to fit the individual patient. The compressed outline of the appliance should fit inside the lingual outline of the teeth. The extended outline shows the amount of preactivation in the appliance

Alternatively the arch width before treatment may be measured using the millimeter scale on the template, measuring the inter-molar width from the gingival margin of the molar and the inter-canine width from the gingival margin of the canines. This distance may be compared with the compressed width and extended width of the transverse appliance on the template to determine the correct size and the range of activation

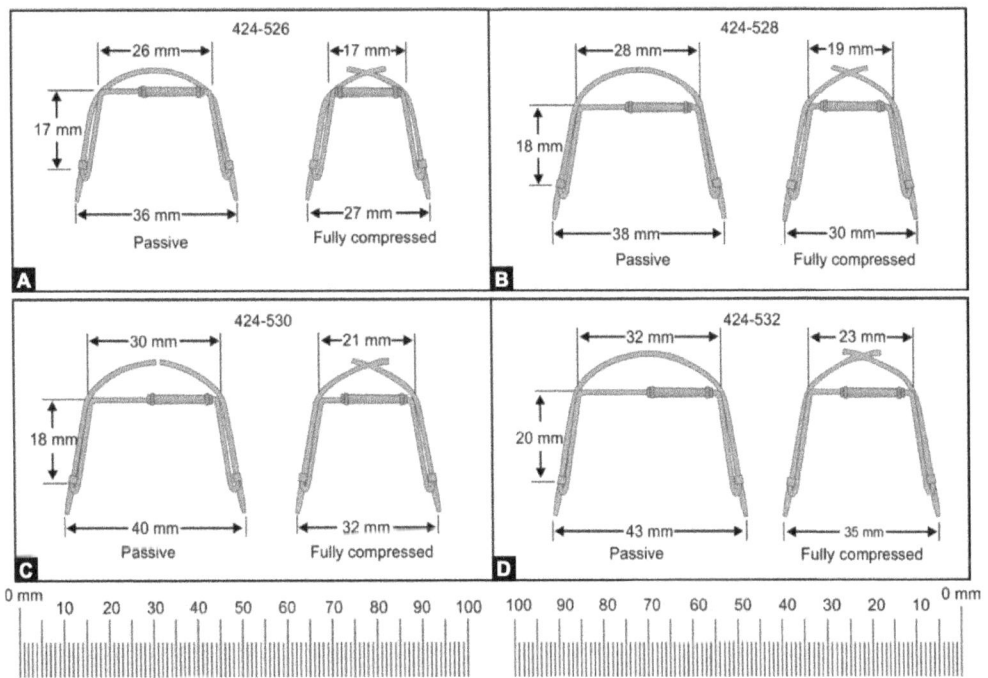

Using the Transverse Template

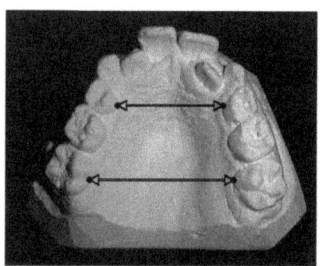

Measure Transverse Width

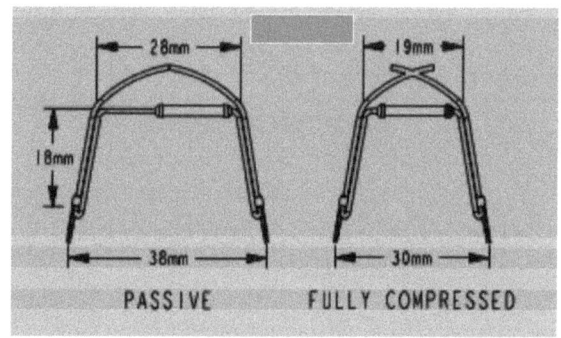

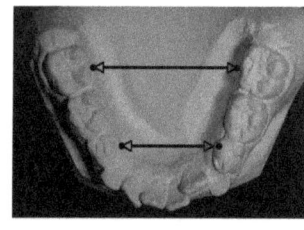

Measure Transverse Width

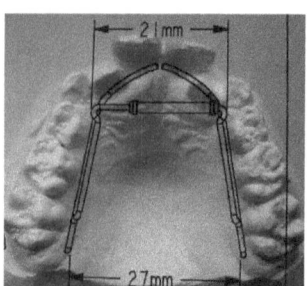

Upper Before & After

The template displays an outline of the appliance in the fully compressed and fully extended size. The correct size is selected by overlaying the image of the appliance on the model. The compressed image must fit inside the arch before treatment. If required the anterior extension wires can be adapted to act on individual teeth. Overlaying the passive image will predict the amount of expansion that will be delivered by the appliance as the compression unit expands.

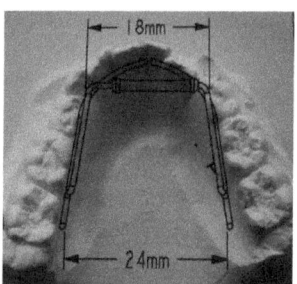

Lower Before & After

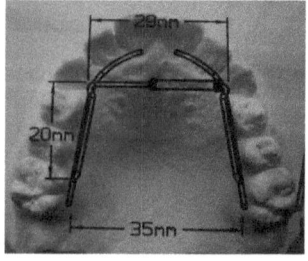

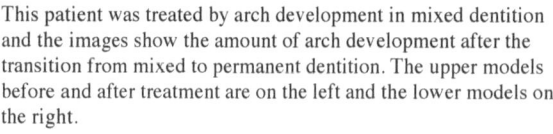

This patient was treated by arch development in mixed dentition and the images show the amount of arch development after the transition from mixed to permanent dentition. The upper models before and after treatment are on the left and the lower models on the right.

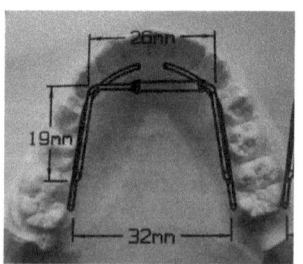

Appliance Fitting

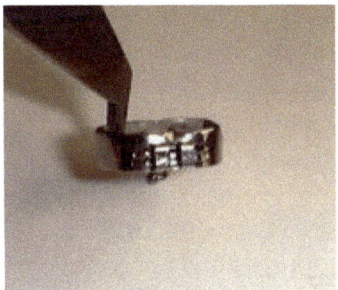

Horizontal Lingual Sheath

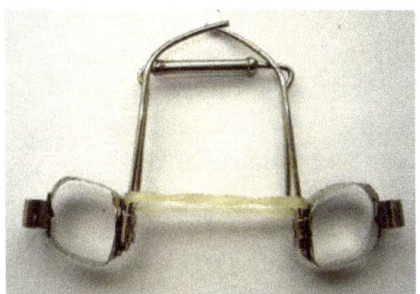

Elastic to facilitate fitting

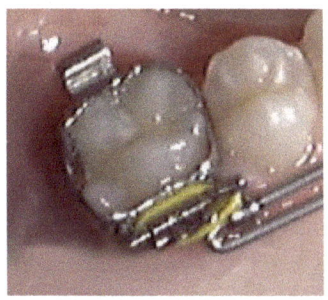

Elastic Tie-back

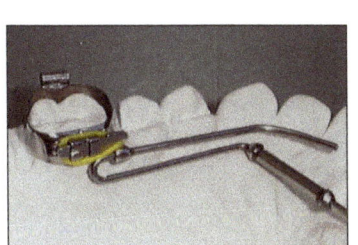

Separators must be placed, preferably within 3 days of the appointment to fit the appliance. The appliance may be prepared on models if an indirect technique is preferred. Molar bands are selected with horizontal lingual sheaths and tried in the mouth to confirm the correct size.

An elastic module is used to compress the Transverse Expander to facilitate appliance fitting. The appliance is fully assembled and is tried in the mouth prior to cementing. Minor adjustment may be required to adapt the appliance to the individual patient.

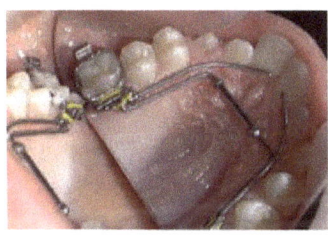

It is easier to attach the molar bands to the lingual wire and fit the appliance in one piece, rather than fitting the bands first then inserting the appliance in the lingual sheaths. An elastic module is used to secure the appliance in the lingual sheath prior to fitting in the mouth. One of the advantages of the TransForce is that it does not occupy the palate. This enables the tongue to adapt into the palate during treatment as the arch expands. In treatment of a constricted maxilla the tongue may adopt a more forward position, which may influence the post pharyngeal airway

TransForce Orthodontics

TransForce Palatal Expander achieves the objective of delivering physiologic forces within the tolerance of the periodontal tissues by applying a light continuous force of 200 grams for maxillary expansion. This approach resolves anterior crowding in mixed or permanent dentition and has the advantage of expanding the lower arch by bony remodeling of the dento alveolar processes. There is equal expansion of the anterior and posterior segments across the inter-canine and inter-molar width.

The compression unit on the TransForce Transverse appliance is positioned lingual to the incisors across the canine region. This is extremely effective in interceptive treatment to resolve upper and lower labial crowding by increasing the intercanine width before the permanent canines erupt. Alternative appliances for palatal expansion are not as effective in correcting anterior crowding. The anterior wires may be used for additional buccal expansion or labial movement of the incisors if required. The arches may be over - expanded in mixed dentition to encourage the premolars and canines to erupt in a wider arch.

In addition to these biological benefits slow expansion techniques offer a number of clinical advantages. An ideal slow expansion appliance requires minimal adjustment throughout its use, but permits easy adjustment when necessary. It delivers a constant physiologic force until the required expansion is obtained. The appliance is light and comfortable enough to be kept in place for sufficient retention of expansion. Prefabrication eliminates extra appointments and the appliance may be selcted and fitted in the laboratory and delivered ready to fit.

TransForce integrates well with fixed appliances in mixed or permanent dentition. Patients should be informed when two phase treatment is planned and it is recommended that brackets are fitted before the anterior teeth are fully aligned from the lingual aspect.

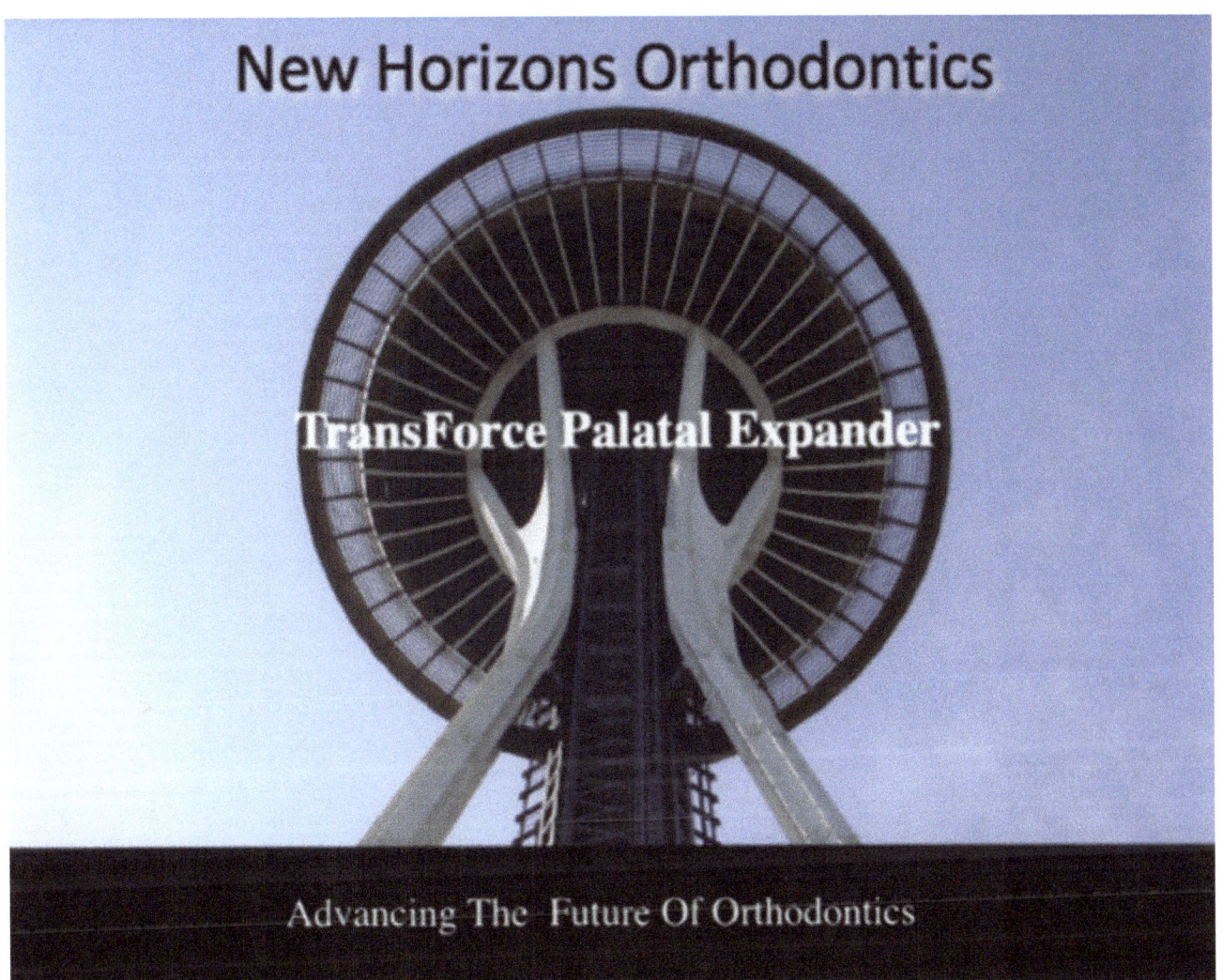

TRANSFORCE PALATAL EXPANDER

Contemporary Treatment Protocol

The protocol for treatment in contemporary orthodontic practice is largely based on a labial approach using prescription bracket systems for correction of malocclusion in permanent dentition. Debate continues within the orthodontic specialty regarding the efficacy of early treatment, and the most advantageous time to commence orthodontic treatment. A lingual approach provides a valid alternative in the management of many malocclusions throughout the age range from early treatment in mixed dentition to effective adult treatment.

Three quarters of facial growth is complete by the age of eight. Primary dentition presents an important phase for treatment of major facial deformities including cleft palate. In the mixed dentition the maxillary and facial sutures are still responsive to adaptive bone growth within the sutures. Arch development techniques play an important part in the management of maxillary contraction by growth modification, whether in primary or mixed dentition. These techniques continue to be effective in the adolescent stage, provided light forces are applied to evoke a physiological response.

Maxillary Arch Development

Maxillary contraction is a common feature in all classes of malocclusion, and is frequently the primary aetiological factor, with secondary effects on the development of the mandible and the lower dental arch .

Consideration of the transverse dimension is important in the efficiency of orofacial functions. The airway may be restricted either in the antero-posterior or transverse dimensions.

A contracted maxilla is of particular significance, in view of its relationship to constriction of the nasal passages, with direct implications for the airway, and this has fundamental effects on general health. Patients with a restricted airway are subject to naso-pharyngeal infection and allergies, and their general health may be adversely affected. (Timms, 1968,1976)

Successful treatment of these conditions is firmly related to early interceptive treatment and is often associated with tooth-size/arch-size discrepancies. (McNamara & Brudon 1983). In many respects this is contrary to the present philosophy of a regimen for orthodontic practice based on treatment in the permanent dentition.

Based on histological studies, the prognosis for treatment of labial segment crowding is better in mixed dentition than in permanent dentition. Melsen (1972) carried out an investigation to determine the histological effect of rapid expansion of the mid-palatal suture in children of various ages. A true stimulation of sutural growth was found only in children who had not attained maximum pubertal growth.

In older individuals expansion resulted in numerous micro-fractures in the sutural region. The post-traumatic reaction around these fractures was of significance for the course of healing, preventing further growth in the suture from taking place.

Development of the maxilla to correct the archform is frequently the first step in treatment to unlock the malocclusion. The maxilla may be contracted antero-posteriorly or transversely, and often in both dimensions, when three-way expansion is indicated. Antero-posterior contraction is characterised by retroclined incisors, as commonly found in Class I bimaxillary retrusion, Class II division 2 and Class III malocclusion.

TREATMENT OF UNILATERAL CROSSBITE IN MIXED DENTITION

An 8 year old girl with a contracted maxilla, resulting in a unilateral crossbite and mandibular displacement to the left on closure requires interceptive treatment by arch development to restore symmetry and improve function in the transition from mixed to permanent dentition

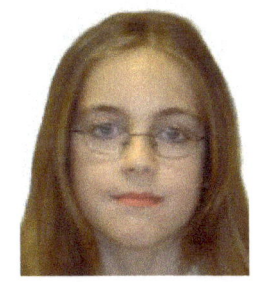
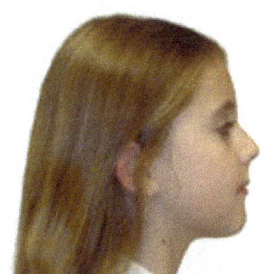

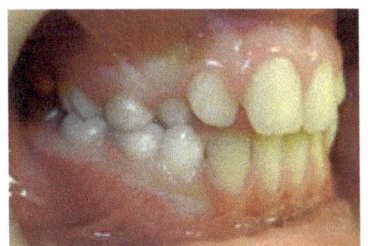
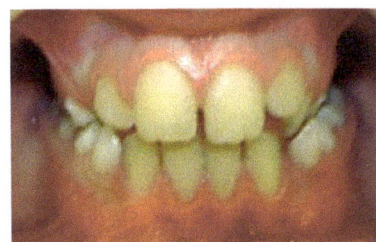
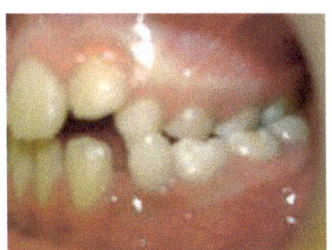

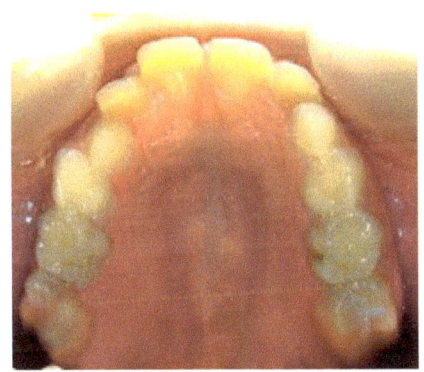
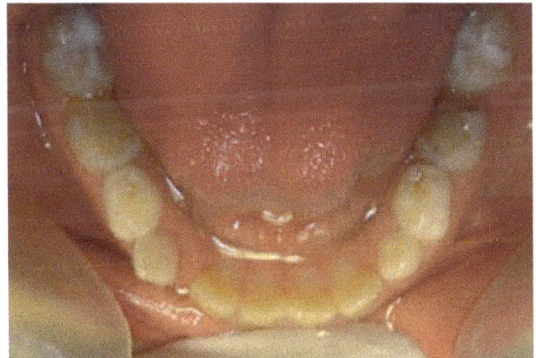

Rapid improvement by maxillary arch development at age 8 years 4 months with a transverse expander corrected the crossbite and improved arch form. After a short period of retention the appliance came loose and was left out. A period of observation followed in the transition to permanent dentition.

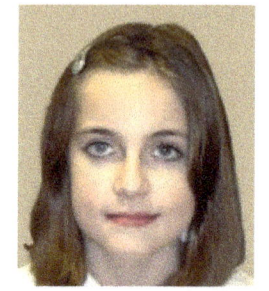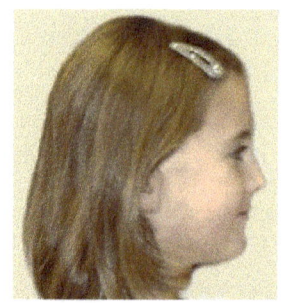

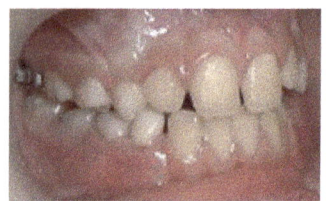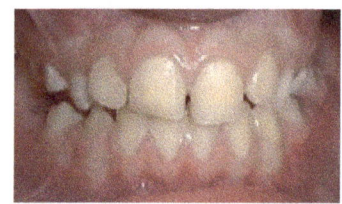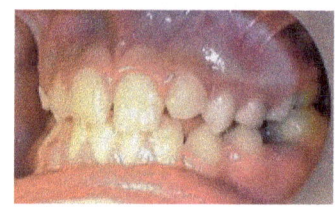

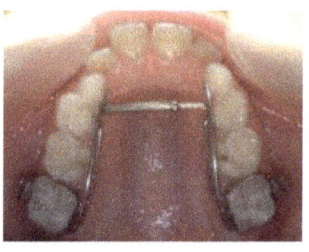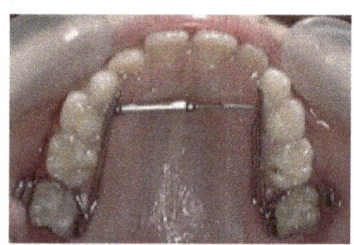

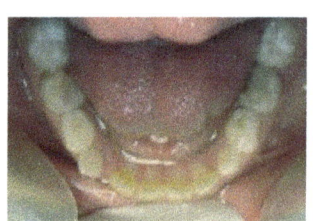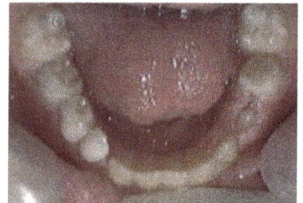

Second Phase

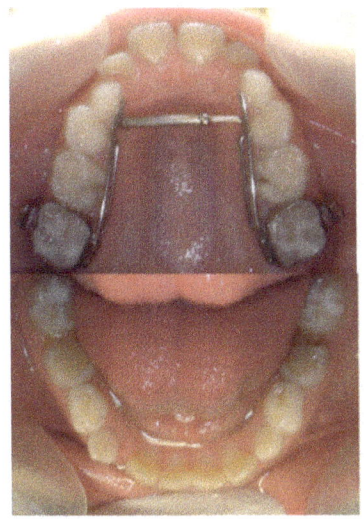 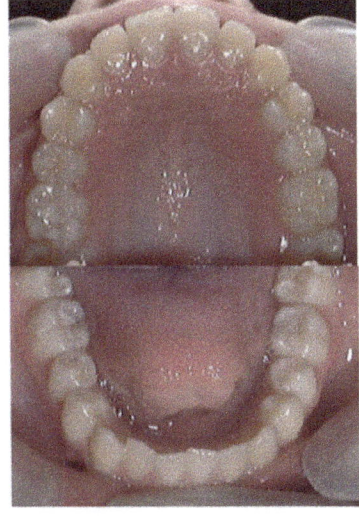

Mixed Dentition   Permanent Dentition

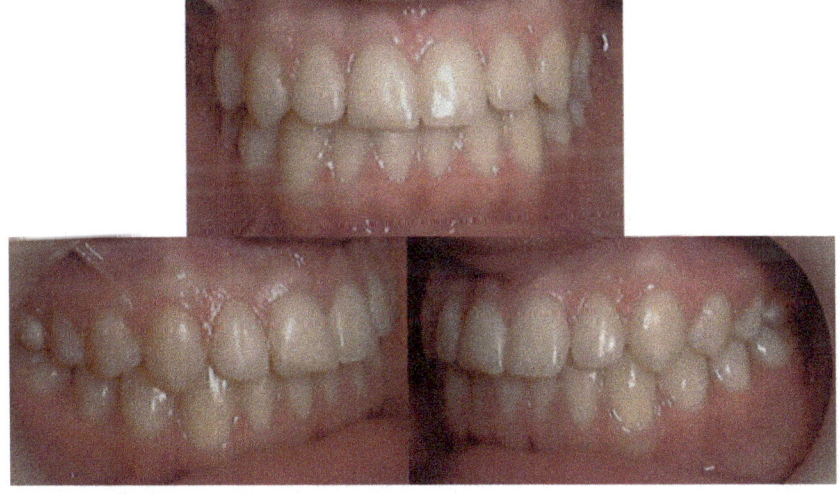

Final photgraphs show the occlusion and arch form at age 12 years 4 months. At this stage the family had move back to England from Portugal and an occlusoguide was fitted as a retainer. to be worn for two hours in the evening and at night to apply pressure to resolve slight lower incisor crowding. This is particularly effective if it is worn when playing computer games, as the patient actively bites into the appliance.

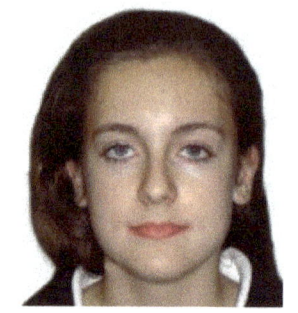 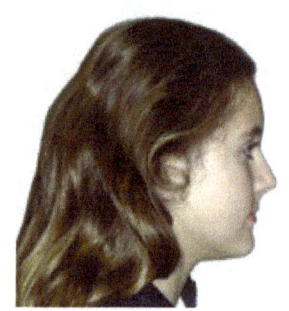

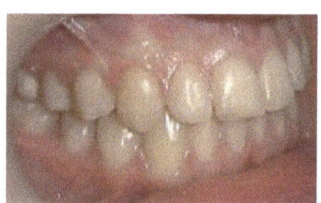 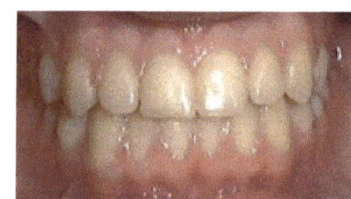 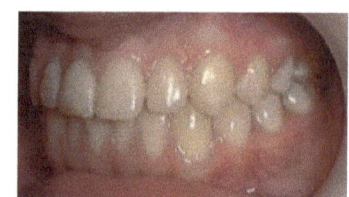

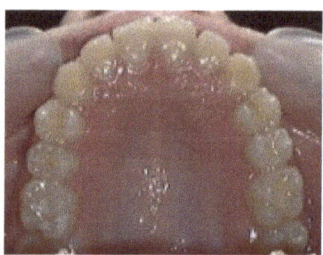 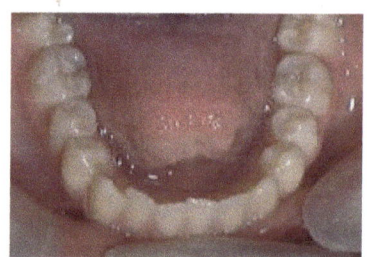

TransForce Orthodontics is equally effective from mixed dentition through to adult therapy

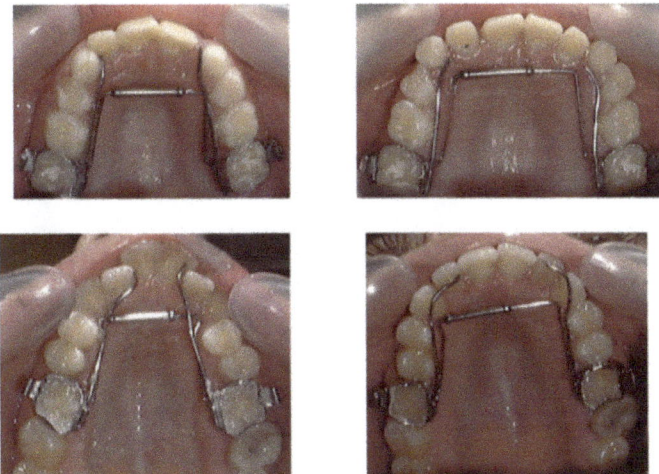

Mixed To Permanent Dentition

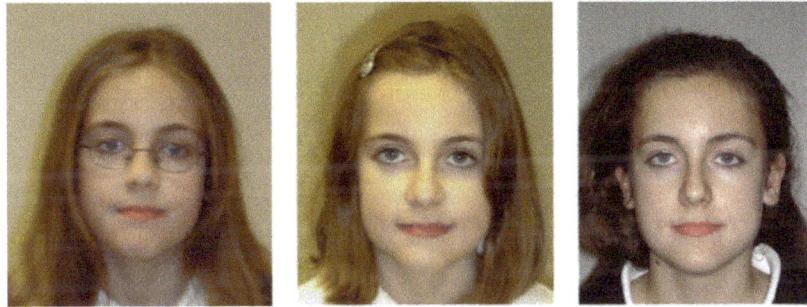

The maxilla is wider after arch development

INTERCEPTIVE TREATMENT OF ANTERIOR CROWDING

A Class III malocclusion with severe upper labial crowding treated in mixed dentition with upper and lower Transforce Transverse Expansion Appliances. Active treatment was completed in 8 months and the Transforce appliances remained in place for 3 months to retain.

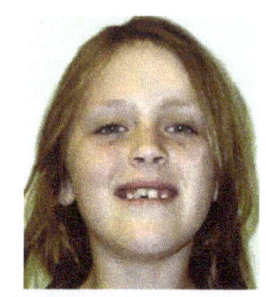

8 Months

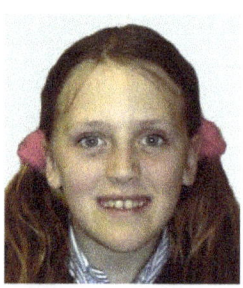

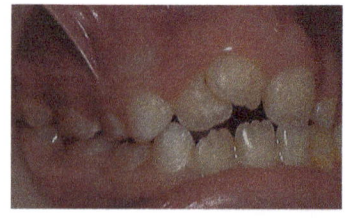

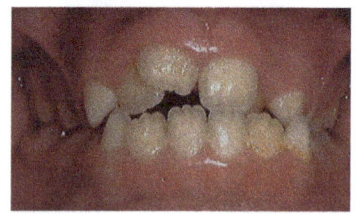

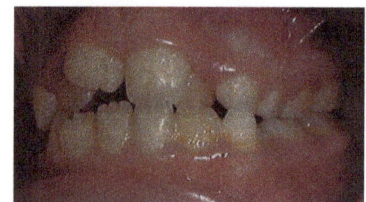

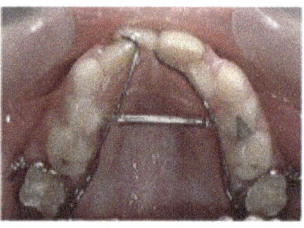

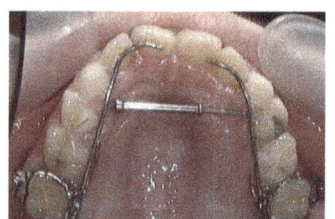

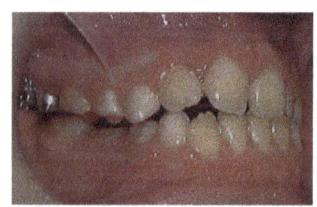

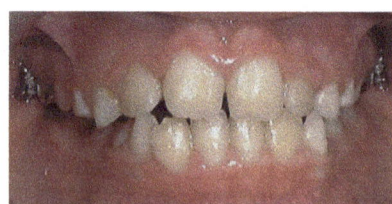

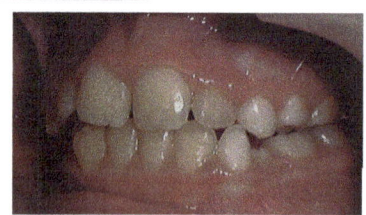

This was followed by a short period of treatment with fixed appliances after eruption of permanent teeth. Interceptive treatment in mixed dentition to resolve anterior crowding simplified the finishing stage and significantly reduced the time required in fixed appliances.

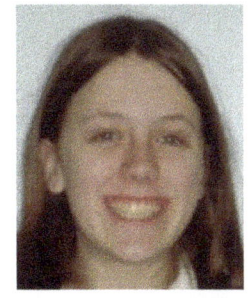 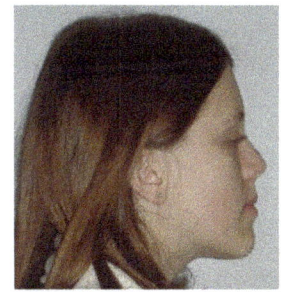

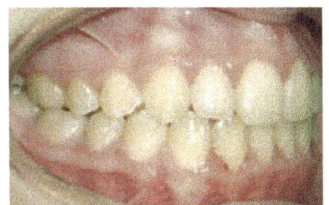 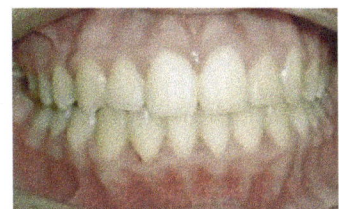 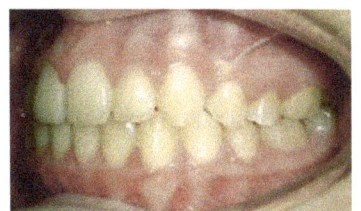

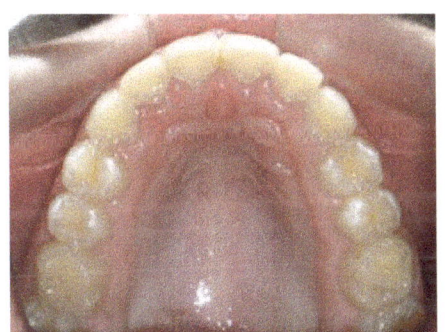 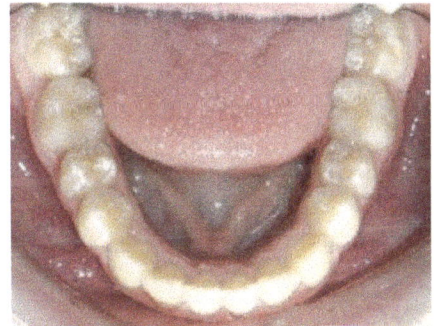

CLASS I CROWDING IN TRANSITIONAL DENTITION

This young boy is approaching the transitional stage from mixed to permanent dentition when he attends for treatment of a bimaxillary dental protrusion with mild crowding in the upper and lower labial segments and lingual occlusion of an upper lateral incisor in a class I malocclusion.

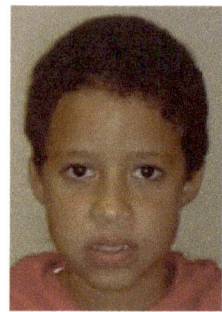
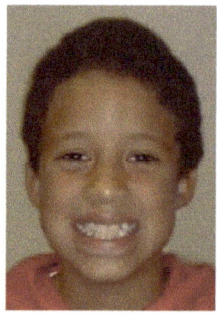
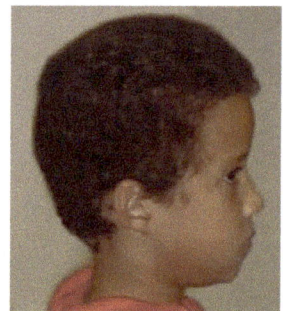

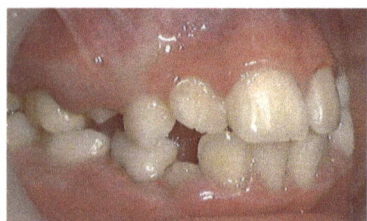
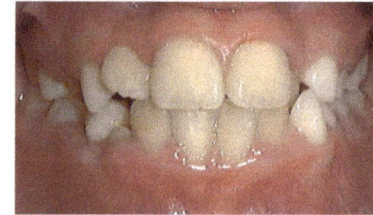
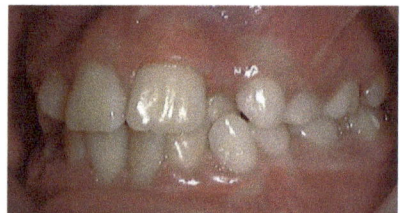

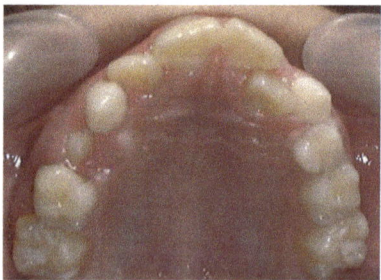
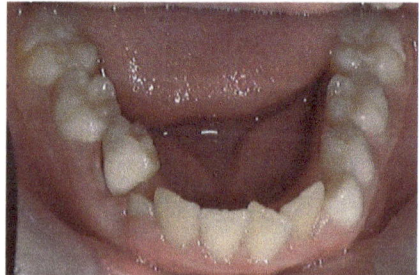

The first step is to expand the arches with Transverse appliances and move the upper lateral incisor distally, and labially. Meantime the first premolars erupt and are obstructed by the TransForce appliance. The appliance is removed to allow the premolars to erupt and then inserted and adapted to move the premolars buccally. After expanding the lower arch a lower fixed appliance is fitted to align the lower labial segment, in combination with the Transforce appliance from the lingual aspect.

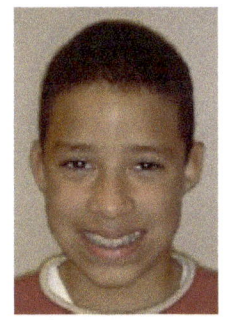
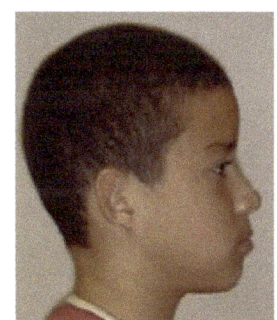

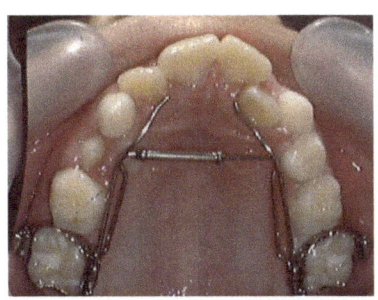
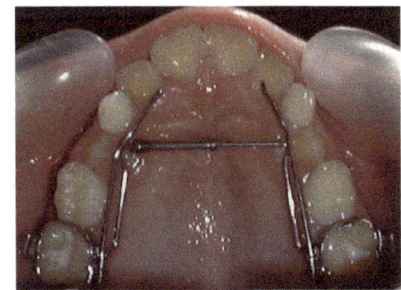
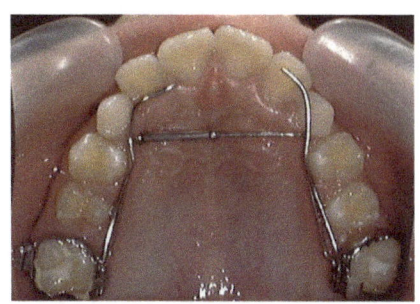

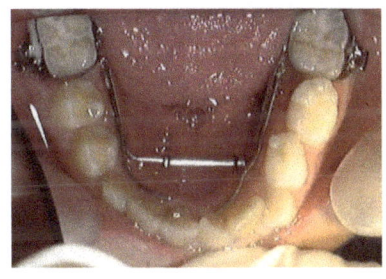
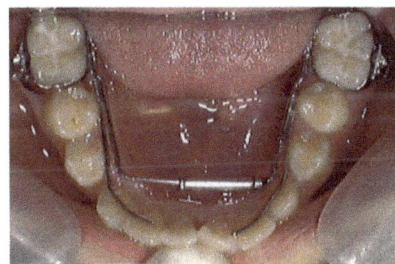
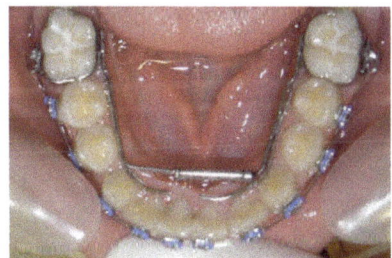

Detailing of the occlusion is completed in 9 months in a finishing stage of treatment with upper and lower fixed appliances.

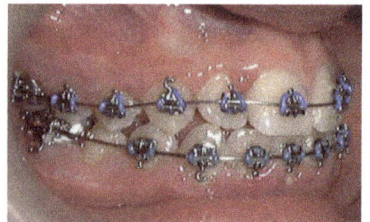
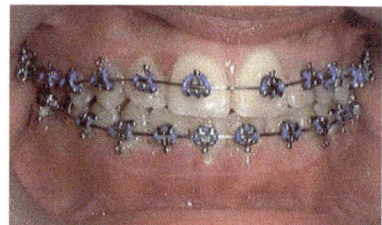
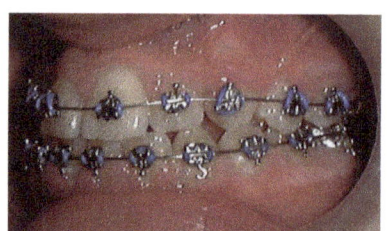

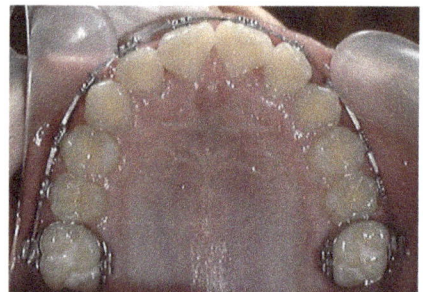
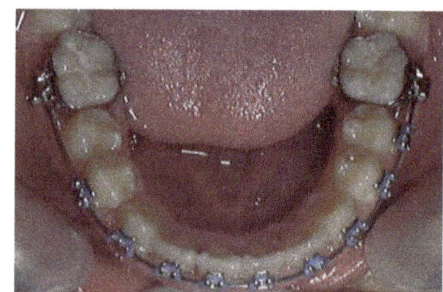

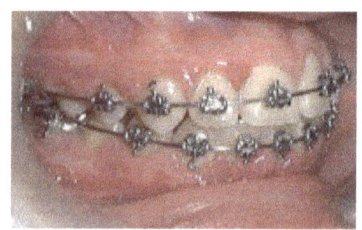
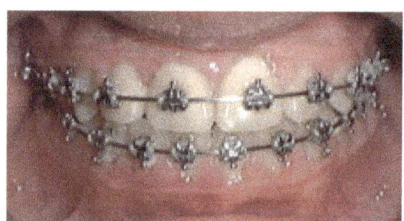
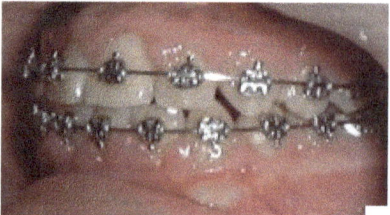

The finished result shows a pleasing profile without extractions. The wide smile and improvement in the facial appearance is in balance with the patient's natural facial type. Interceptive treatment by arch development in the transitional dentition simplified the management of this malocclusion

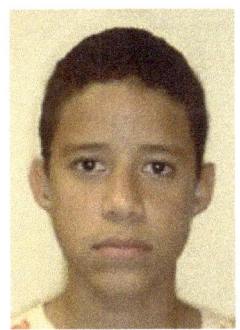 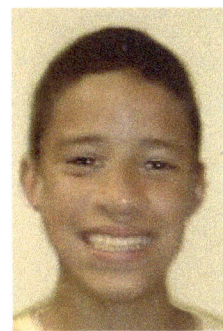 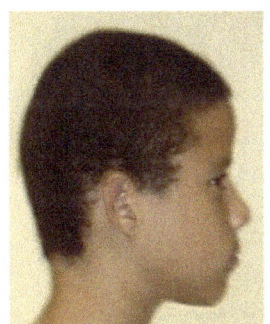

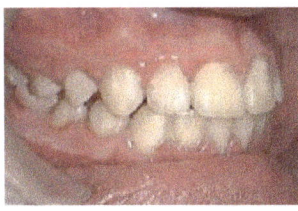 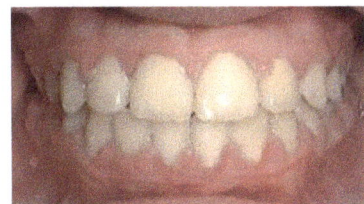 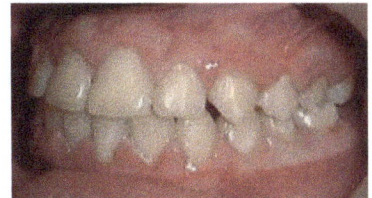

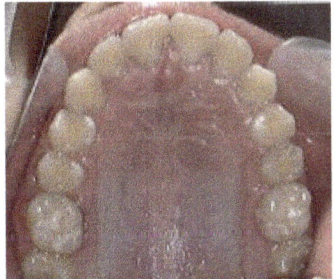 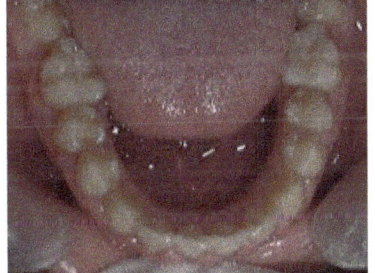

LABIAL SEGMENT CROWDING IN CLASS II DIVISION 2 MALOCCLUSION

Maxillary contraction is responsible for labial segment crowding with a lateral incisor completely blocked out of the arch at age 10 years 6 months. Gingival recession of a lower incisor is due to traumatic occlusion with four lower incisors trapped by three retroclined upper incisors. Transverse arch development is required to unlock the malocclusion.

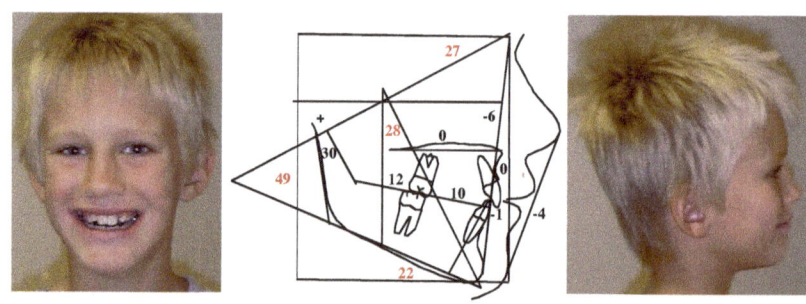

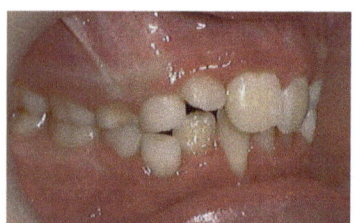
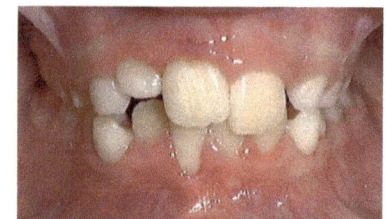
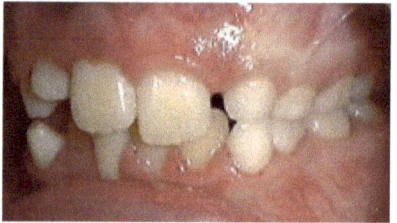

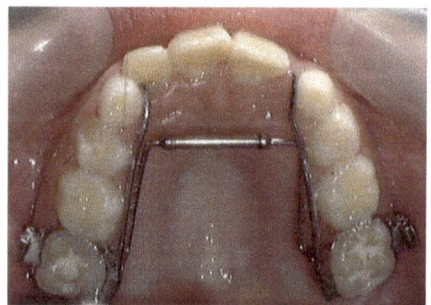
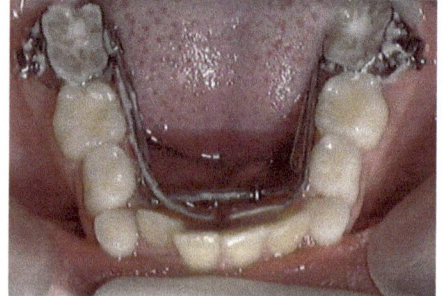

TransForce Transverse expansion appliances are used to over-correct arch width in the mixed dentition This successfully accommodates the lateral incisor and relieves the traumatic occlusion on the lower incisors. In treating a crowded lower labial segments it is important to guide the lower canines to erupt in a wider arch to increase the intercanine width. Over-correction of deciduous molars aims to encourage their permanent successors to erupt buccally to improve the archform.

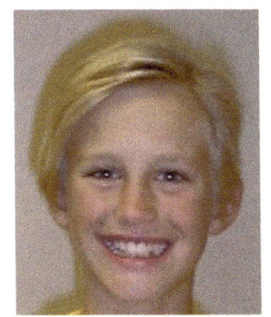 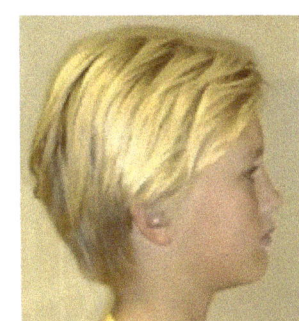

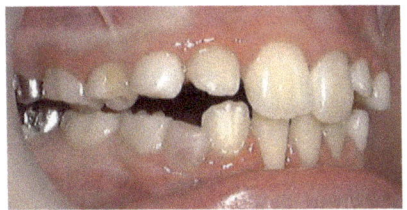 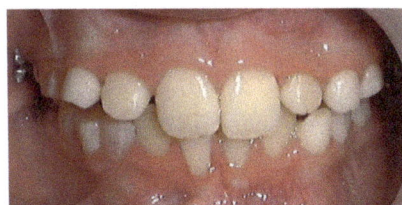 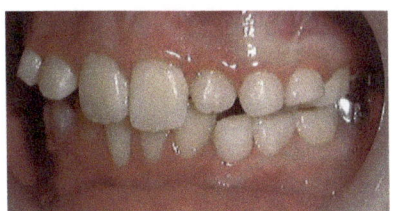

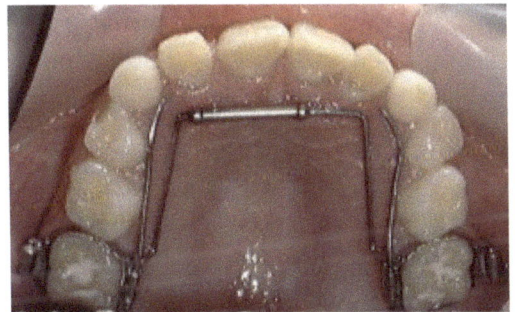 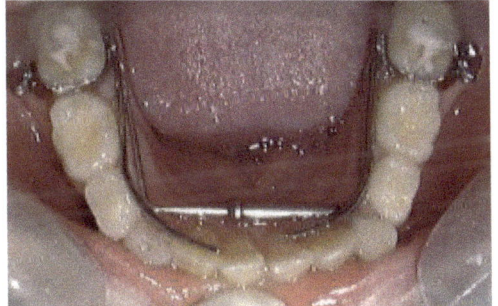

TransForce Sagittal Expander is designed to increase arch length by applying light physiologic forces to advance the anterior teeth. It is indicated when the incisors are retroclined with deep overbite for patients with a flat profile or bimaxillary retrusion. Reciprocal forces are applied to the molars and the anterior teeth and the force levels favour labial movement of the anterior teeth.

Molar width increases as the sagittal appliance expands due to the angulation of the compresion units. Addditional transverse expansion may be acheived by activating the anterior extension wires to move premolars and canines or deciduous teeth buccally if required. This may be indicated in mixed dentition to over expand the arch in order to encourage premolars and canines to erupt in a wider arch.

Correction of Dental Asymmetry

The Transforce Sagittal Expander is extremely effective at correcting dental asymmetry by equalizing the space available for eruption of premolars and canines on each side. When the appliance is inserted it is more compressed on the side that has more crowding and as it expands it corrects the asymmetry and accommodates the erupting teeth on both sides. This is effective in both arches and it is a unique advantage of the pre-activated Transforce Sagittal Expander that does not apply to any other appliance.

In conclusion this report outlines the advantages of pre-activated Transverse and Sagittal TransForce appliances compared to alternative appliance systems for palatal and lingual expansion in both dental arches. TransForce Orthodontics delivers three way expansion and is effective from mixed dentition through adolescence to adult therapy in all classes of malocclusion.

After arch development the TransForce appliances remained in place to retain the position until the lateral incisor erupted. This allowed the centre line to correct and the gingival condition improved on the lower incisors. C/C width settled to 28 mm from original of 21 mm and 6/6 width increased from 31 to 38 mm. Lower molar width increased from 30 to 36 mm. Visits were less frequent and appliances were left out while premolars and canines erupted. This patient was a goalkeeper and preferred not to have an upper fixed appliance. Treatment was completed with upper & lower sagittal TransForce appliances supported by a lower fixed appliance.

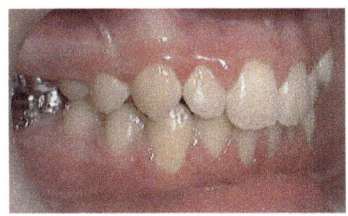 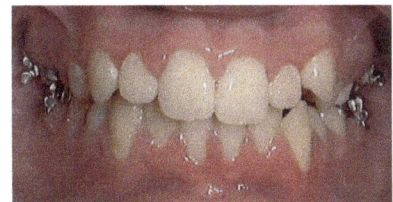 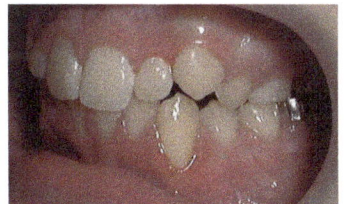

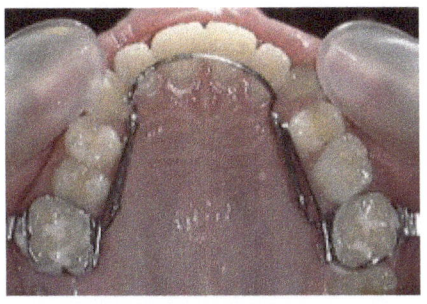 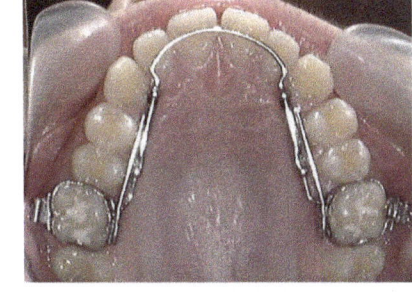

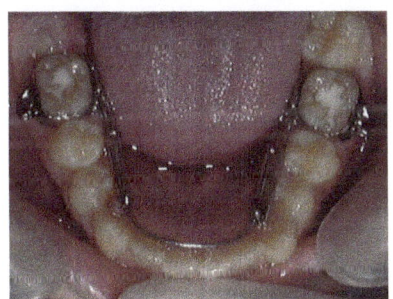 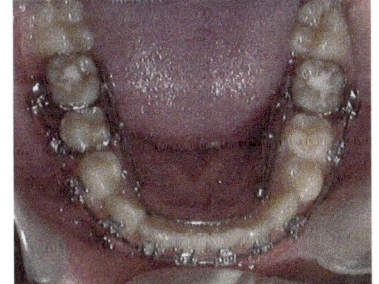

TRANSVERSE & SAGITTAL ARCH DEVELOPMENT IN CLASS II MALOCCLUSION

This patient presented a Class II Division I malocclusion with a narrow 'V' shaped upper arch and a crowded lower arch. He was unwilling to have fixed appliances, but was happy to wear invisible lingual appliances. An upper Transverse appliance was fitted first to widen the upper arch and provide space to align the collapsed lower labial segment.

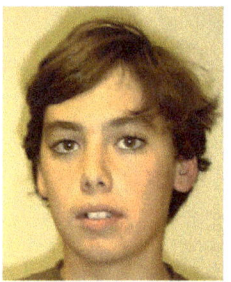 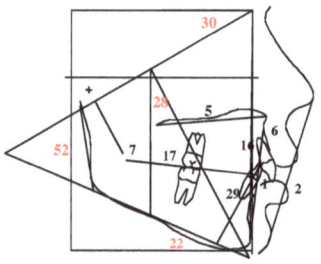 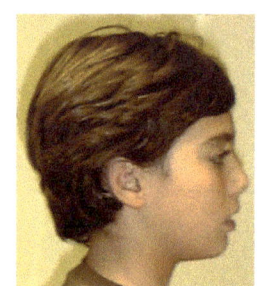

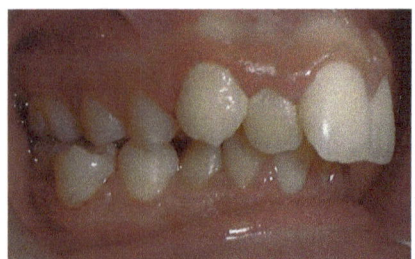 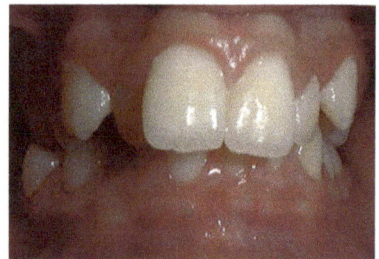 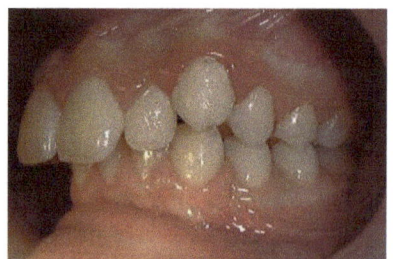

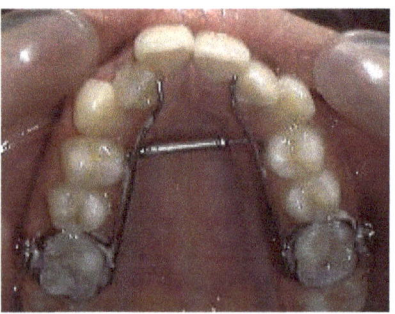 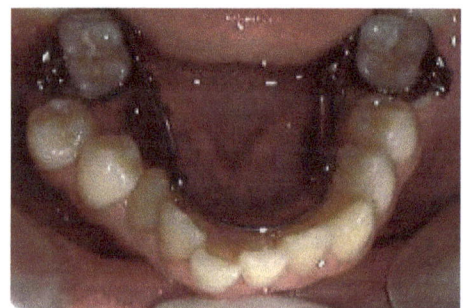

Creating space by transverse expansion of the upper arch increased upper inter-canine width and freed the lower arch for sagittal and transverse development. This unlocked the occlusion and allowed a lower sagittal appliance to be fitted two months later to improve the lower arch form. The following photographs show the progress on the third visit after 4 months of maxillary expansion. As treatment progressed the patient agreed to have a lower fixed appliance fitted to improve control and stability in the lower arch.

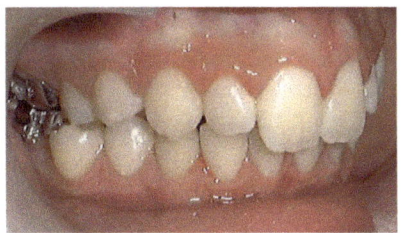 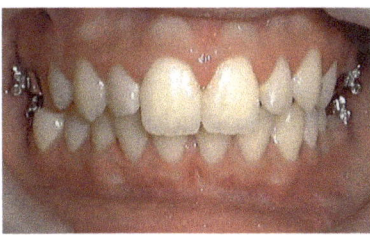 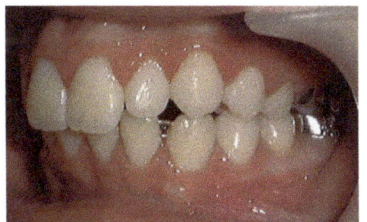

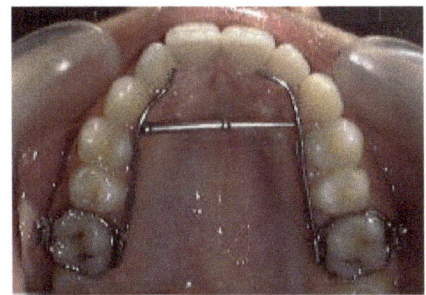 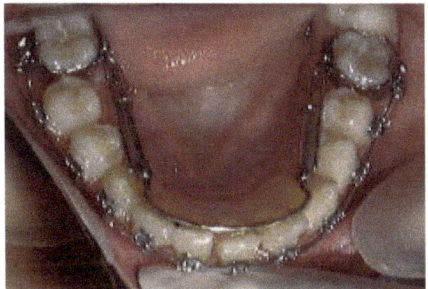

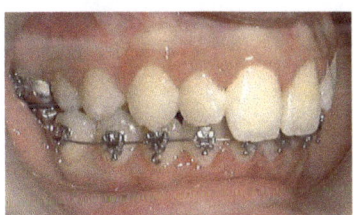 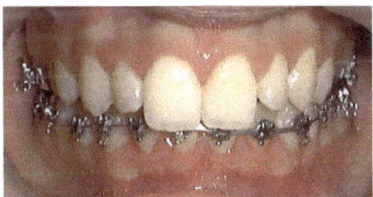 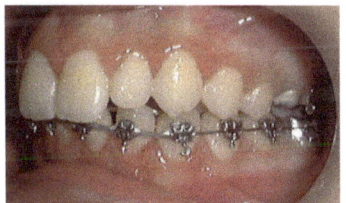

This severe malocclusion was not treated to an ideal result, as the patient requested early removal of appliances. A marked improvement was achieved with simple appliances followed by retainers and treatment was completed in 8 visits over a period of 16 months followed by retainers.

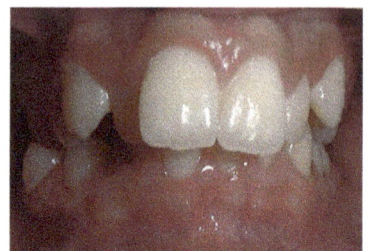 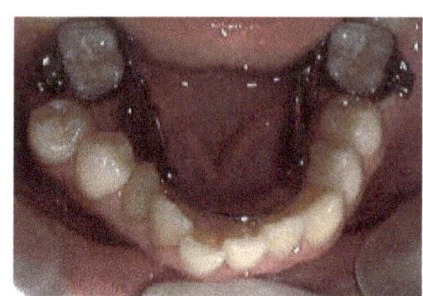

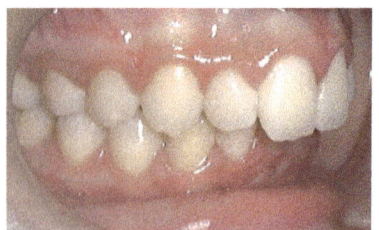 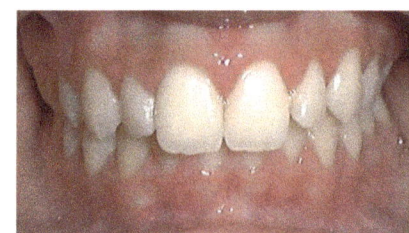 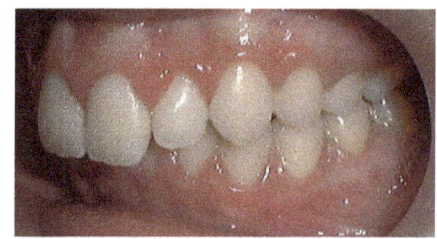

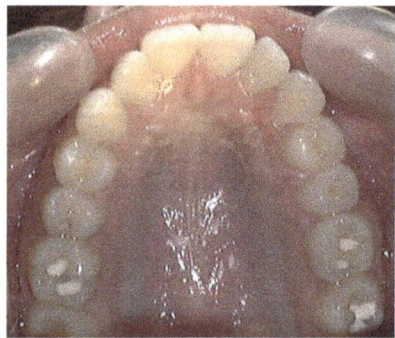 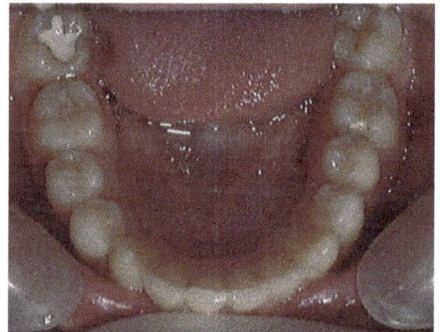

Transverse & Sagittal Arch Development

Occlusion Before Treatment

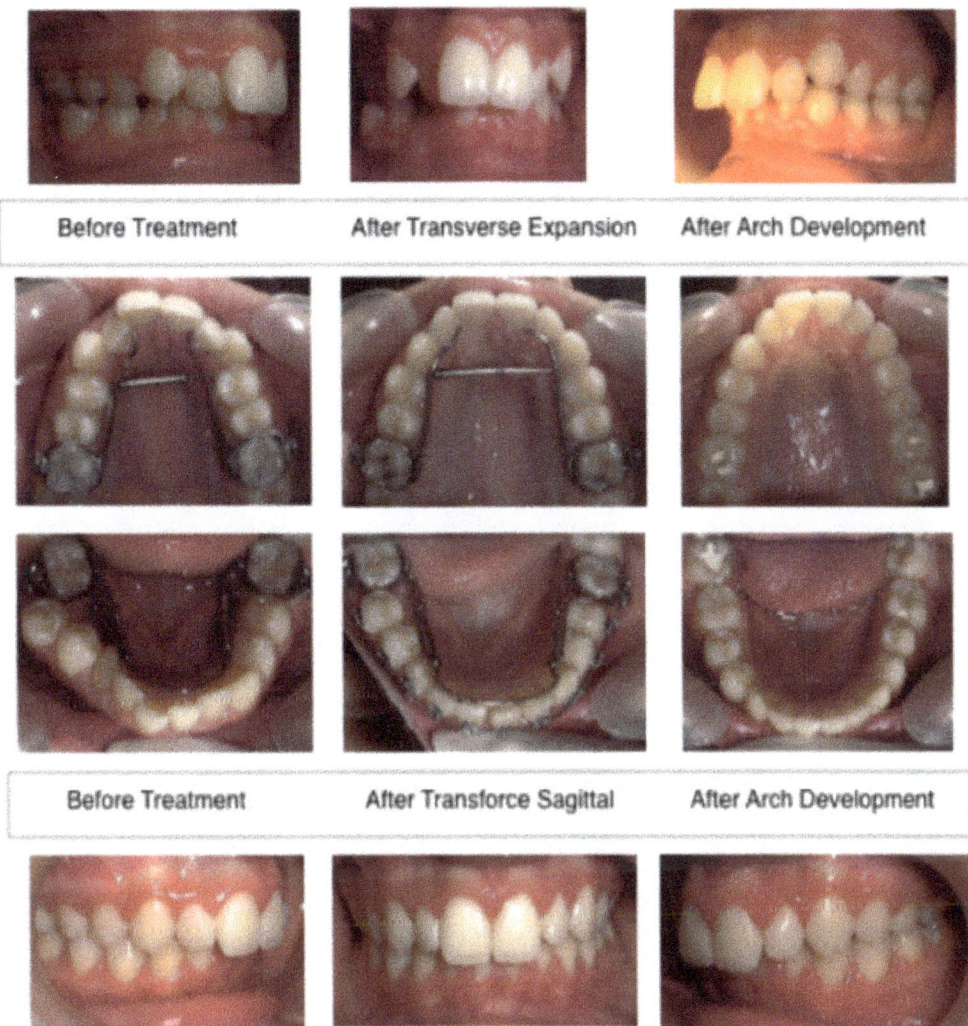

Before Treatment | After Transverse Expansion | After Arch Development

Before Treatment | After Transforce Sagittal | After Arch Development

TRANSVERSE DEVELOPMENT IN DOLICHOFACIAL PATTERN

A 12 year old with a narrow maxilla and severe upper labial crowding in a severe dolichofacial pattern presents a challenge to accommodate a lateral incisor, which is blocked out of the arch lingually. A TransForce transverse expander is fitted and within four months has created space for the displaced incisor, with the additional benefit that the upper canine has spontaneously moved distally as the incisor is advanced. The upper fixed appliance is fitted at the this visit with a lower transverse appliance to expand the lower arch without advancing the incisors. This is followed by a lower fixed appliance and treatment is completed in 18 months.

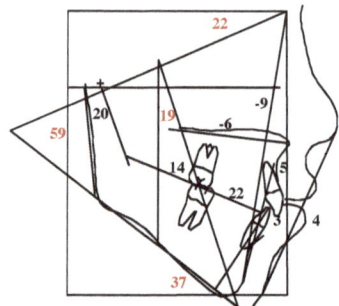

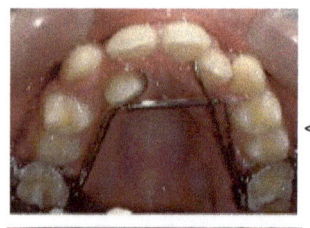
4 Months
<======>
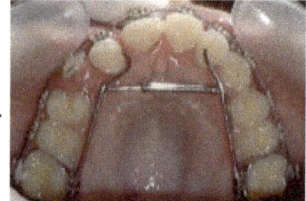
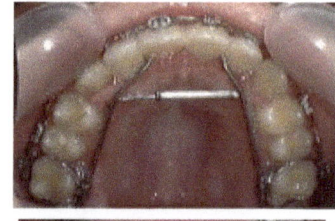

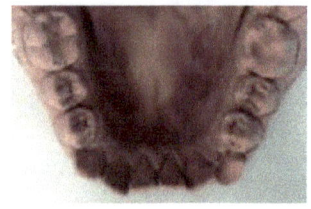
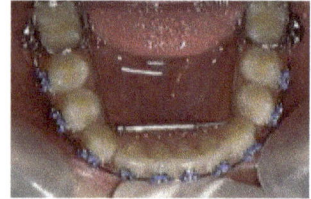
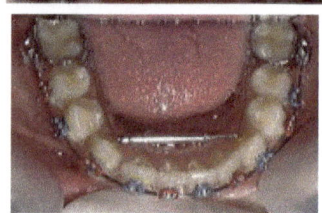

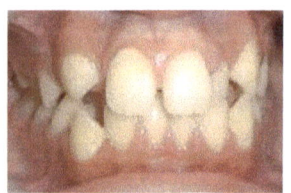
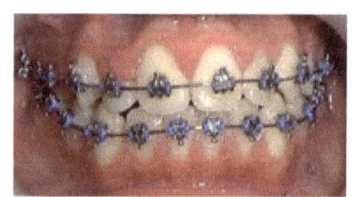
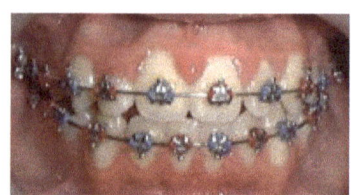

At age 14 the lips were incompetent and formed an oral seal with difficulty. Removable retainers were fitted and worn for 14 months before leaving it out to observe the response. The lateral incisor moved lingually a little and a quad helix was fitted for 8 months to align and support this tooth, followed by a fixed lingual retainer.

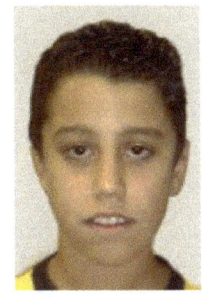
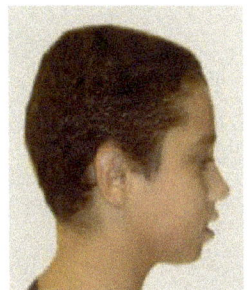
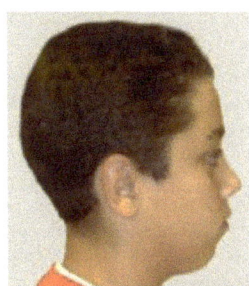

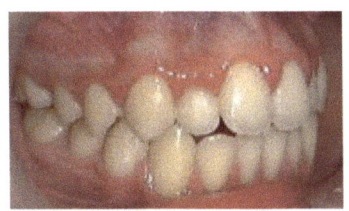
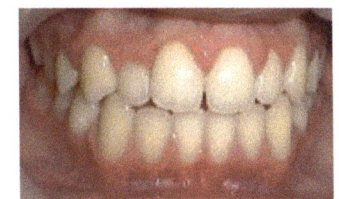
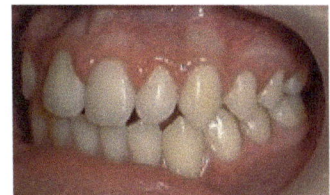

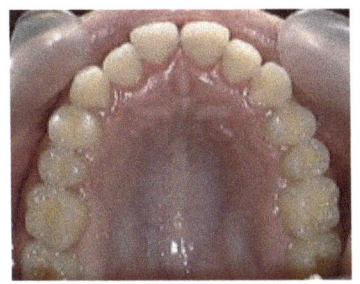
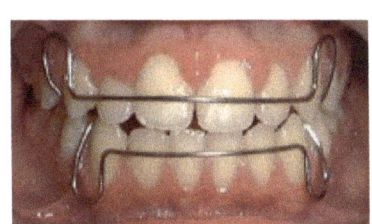
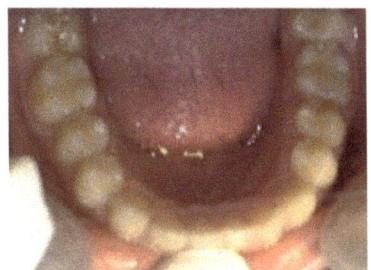

The patient returned at age 21, when his lingual retainer came out. Although his oral hygiene had lapsed the occlusion was stable and there appeared to be no need for further retention. The dolichofacial pattern has not changed, but maturation of oro-facial musculature has improved the lip seal and facial balance is restored.

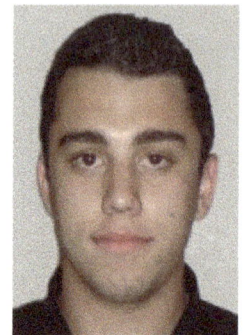 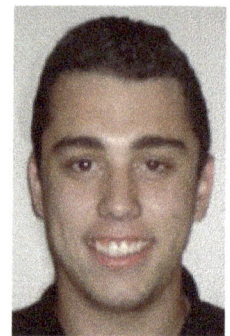 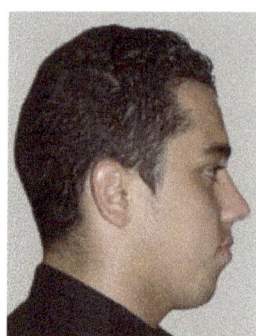

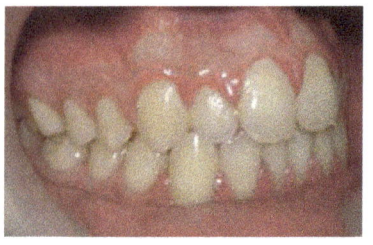 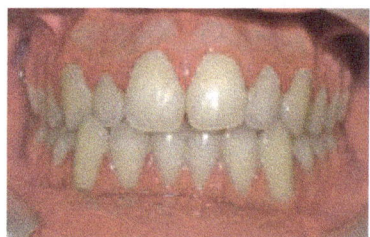 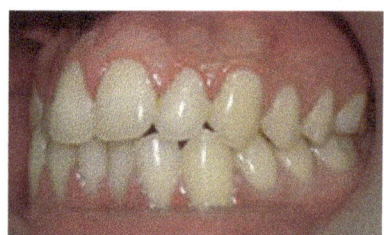

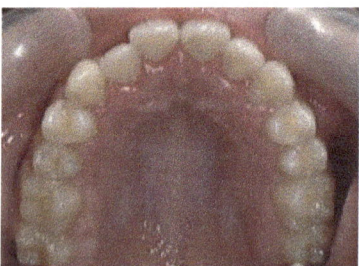 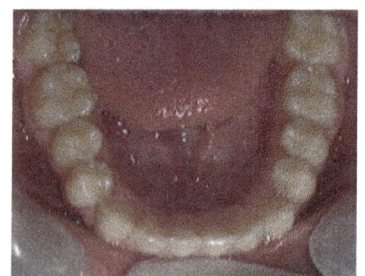

ARCH DEVELOPMENT IN ADULT THERAPY

This young adult prefers to have invisible appliances. She presents severe maxillary contraction with labial segment crowding, crossbite of /4, and lingual occlusion of lateral incisors. Upper molars are rotated into crossbite. A transverse expander must be adapted to fit in lingual sheaths on the molars and is adjusted during treatment to correct the molar rotation and expand inter-molar width.

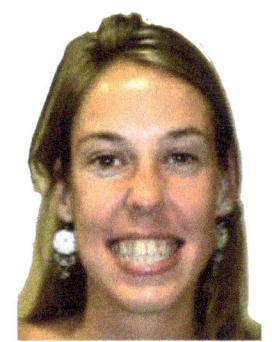 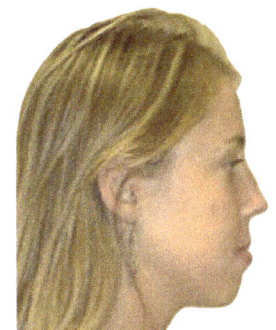

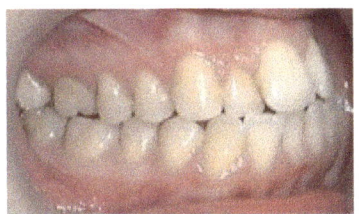 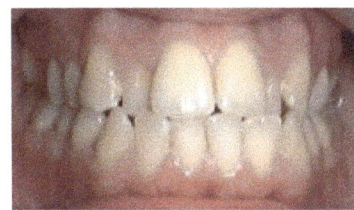 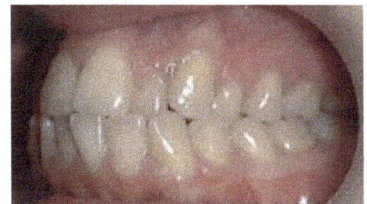

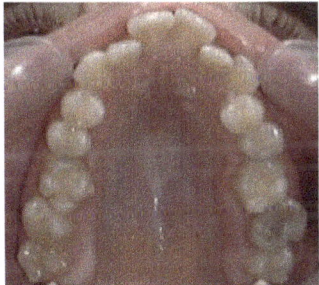 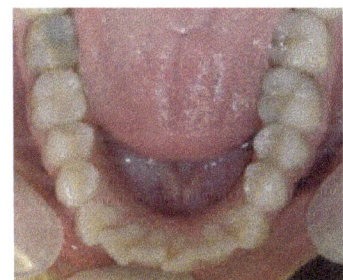

This patient's smile noticeably improved after 4 months and she enjoyed having invisible appliances for 11 months before progressing to a short period with aesthetic fixed appliances to complete treatment. These records show the changes in facial appearance in 8 months and improvement in archform in 11 months with a *TransForce* appliance.

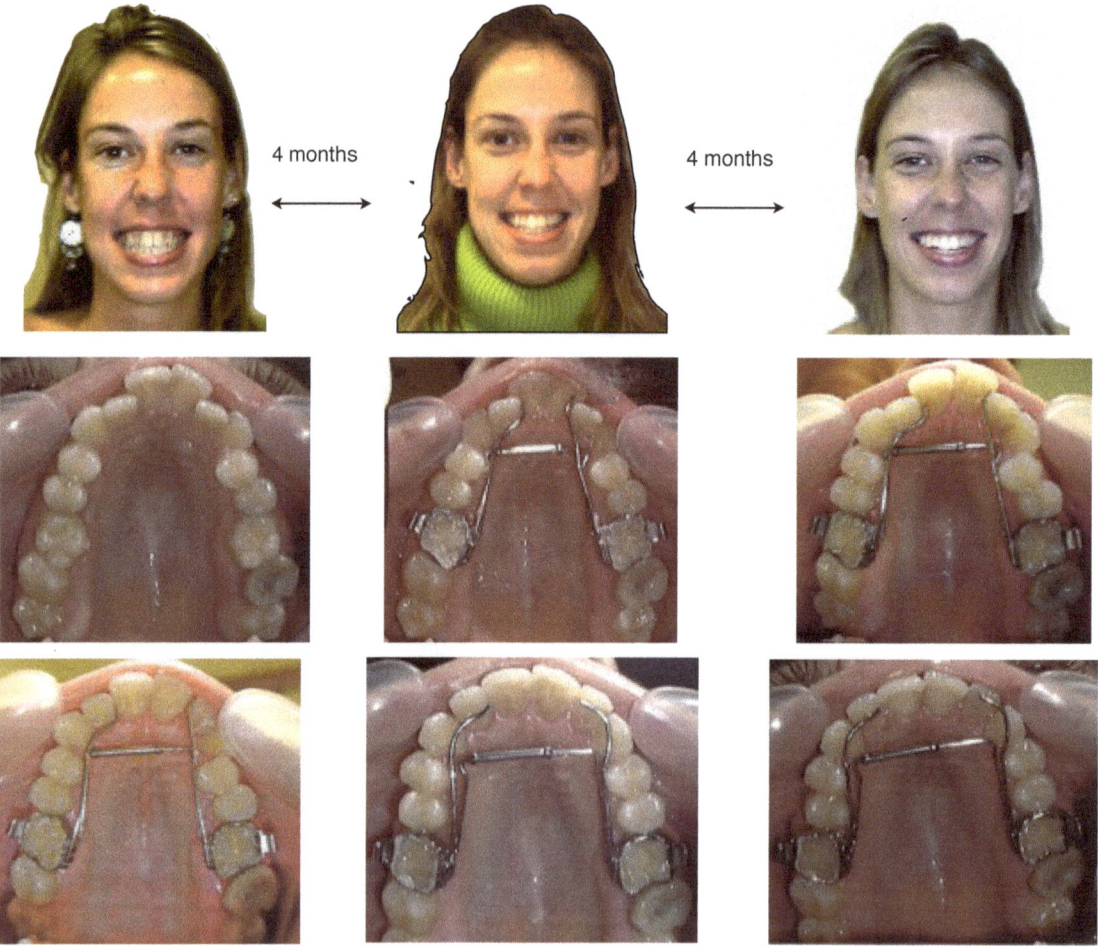

The upper and lower anterior teeth are aligned by gentle pressure from the lingual aspect before brackets are placed.
A lower fixed appliance is fitted after 8 months, and upper brackets after 11 months. The period in full bonded appliances is reduced to 12 months in the lower arch and 9 months in the upper arch.

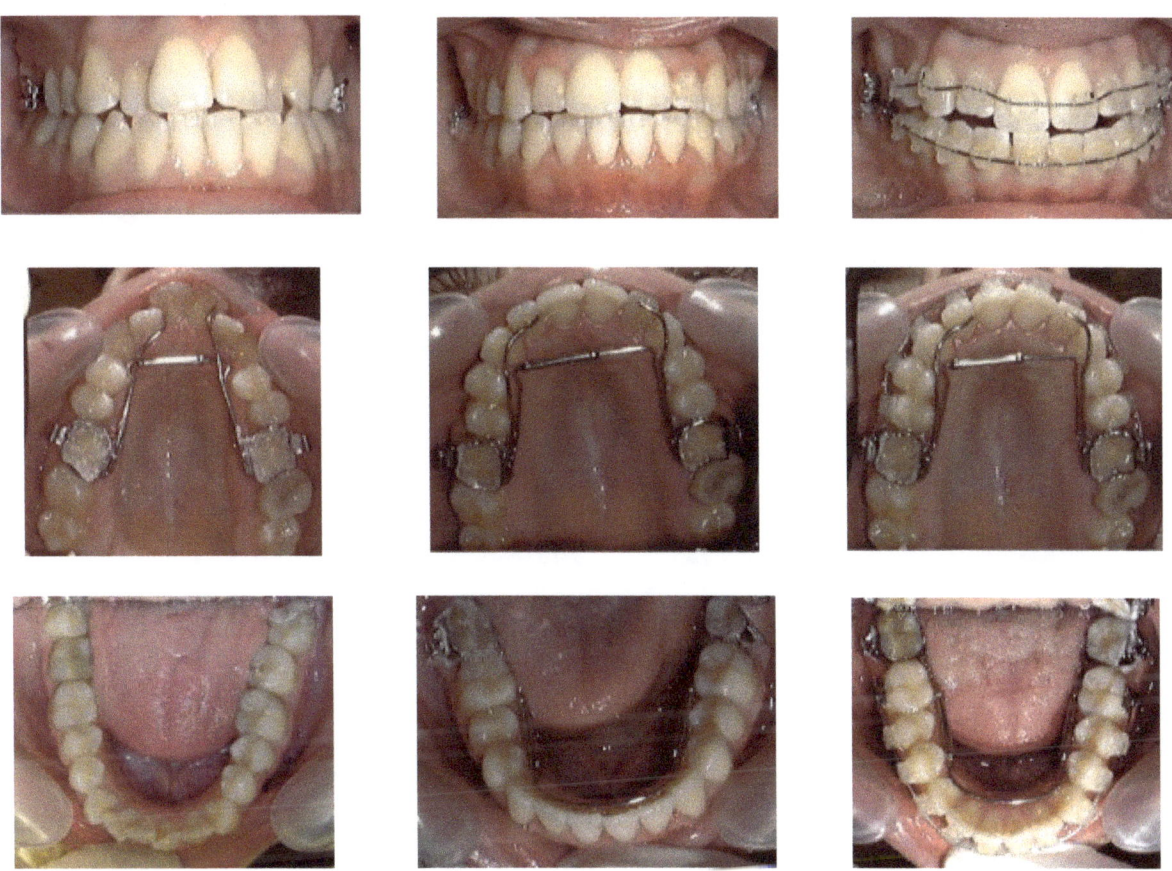

A customized upper utility expansion arch was used to advance the upper incisors and Class III inter-maxillary elastics were worn for for 4 months to correct the lingual occlusion. During this time the overjet was over-corrected to 5 mm to allow for rebound, and the appliances were removed at this visit, while retention continued with the TransForce appliance.

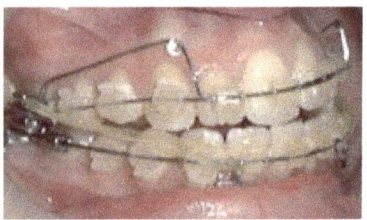 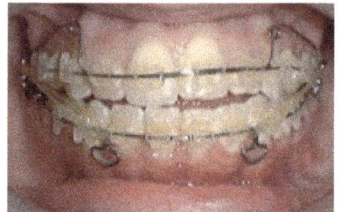 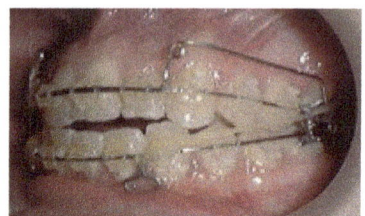

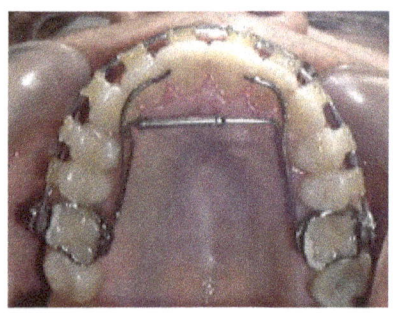 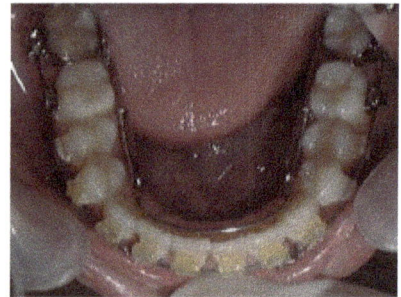

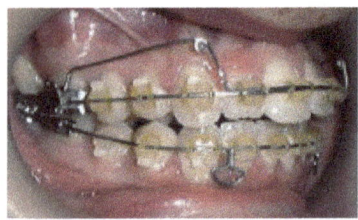 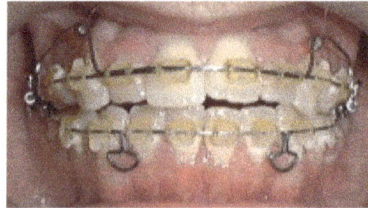 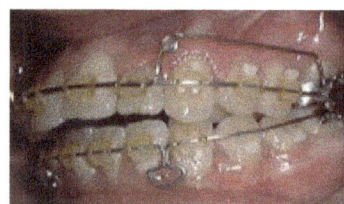

During the early stages of treatment extraction of a lower incisor or lower premolars was considered to create space to retract the lower anterior teeth to correct the incisor relationship and improve the profile. However the patient's dentist carried out the unplanned extraction of lower third molars and this changed the treatment plan. It was decided to continue to develop the lower arch and a lower sagittal appliance was fitted in second molar bands to attempt to move these teeth distally and gain a little space to retract the incisors by applying Class III elastics. After treatment the upper and lower TransForce appliances were used as retainers initially to allow the occlusion to settle before fitting fixed lingual retainers.

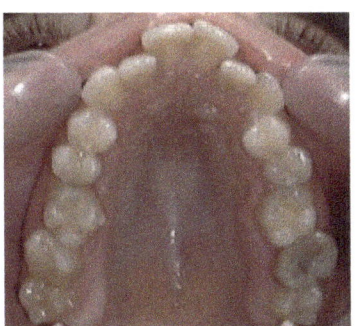
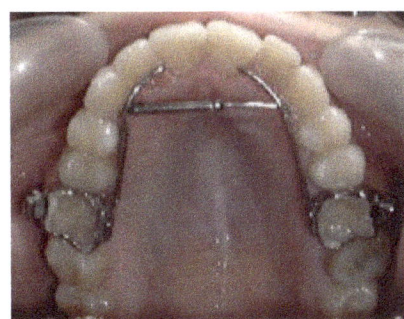
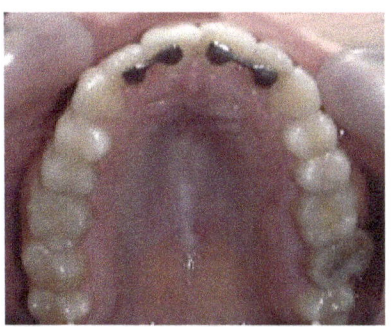

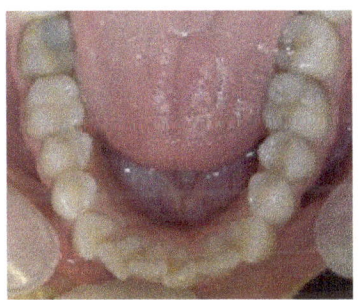
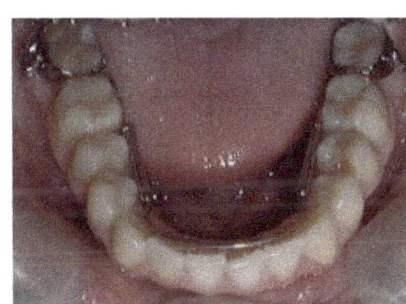
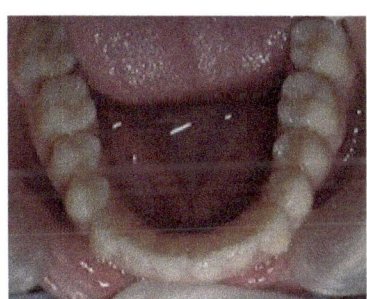

The lingual approach presents minimum discomfort and inconvenience for adults. Invisible lingual appliances simplify treatment using biocompatible forces for gentle arch development. Typically the time in fixed appliances is reduced by 50%. Treatment was completed in 19 months and bonded fixed appliances were worn for less than half the treatment time.

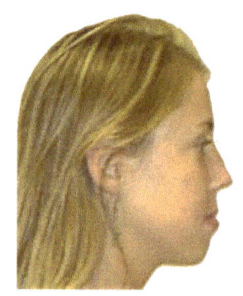 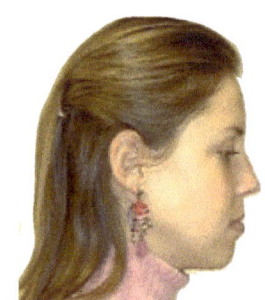

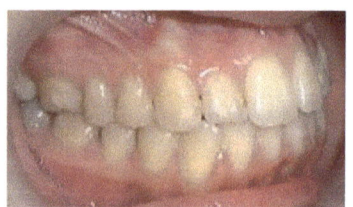 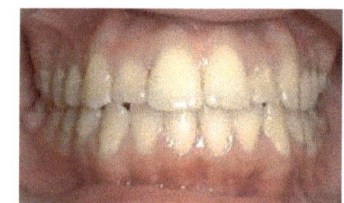 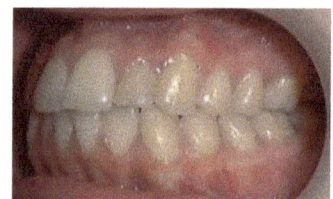

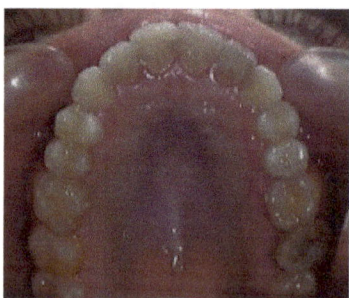 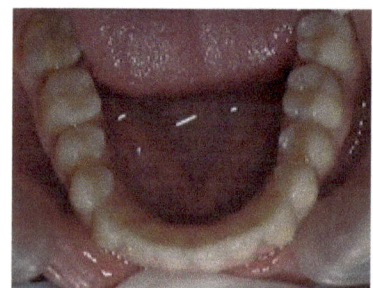

Cranial Base Angle 30°: Facial Axis 26°: Mandibular Plane 31° Convexity 1 mm

In a growing patient a dolichofacial Class III pattern always presents a challenge so it is an advantage to treat this problem when the patient is no longer growing. An increased cranial base angle combined with a high mandibular plane angle accounts for the increased facial height, and mandibular growth has compensated skeletally to produce a straight profile. The lower incisor is 9 mm ahead of the A-Po line and this accounts for the prominent lower lip. Treatment is successful in retracting the lower dentition and this improves the profile.

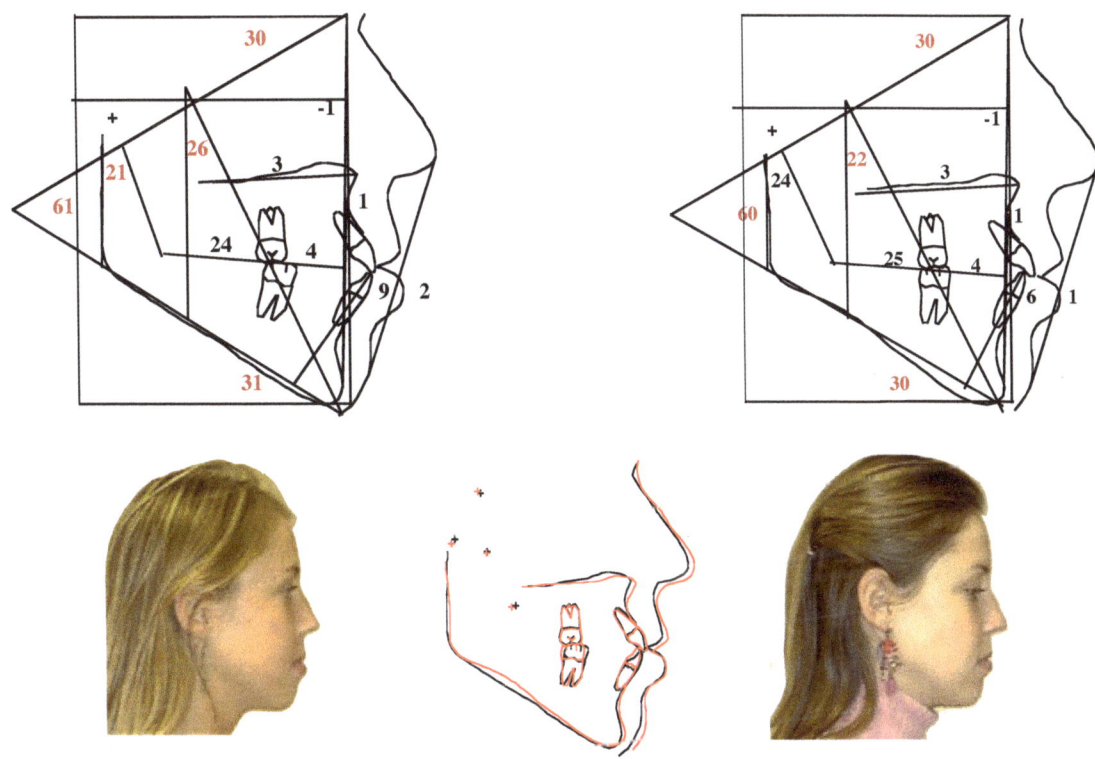

43

Appliance Removal and Retention

Transforce appliances are normally left in situ to act as a retainer after activation is complete. After sagittal correction arch development may be followed by bonded fixed appliances for detailed finishing. The lingual appliance may be integrated with fixed appliances, or alternatively it can be removed by compressing the coil spring to remove the wire tags from the molar sheaths.

After transverse development a period of retention encourages the tongue to adapt into the expanded palate and the altered tongue position then helps to stabilize the arch form after removal of appliances. The Transverse Expander is easily integrated with fixed appliances, and may remain in place to retain the arch width during subsequent treatment. Alternatively it may be removed from the molar sheaths after appropriate retention of the transverse dimension.

Advantages of Transforce Lingual Appliances

Transforce appliances significantly reduce chair time in treatment of many malocclusions. Slow steady development of arch form using light continuous forces does not cause discomfort. The patient benefits aesthetically by using invisble appliances for half the time in treatment. Appointments are less frequent during arch development.

Typically the period of treatment with bonded fixed appliances is reduced by 50 %. This benefits both the patient and the orthodontist, providing a treatment protocol that is compatible in modern society by reducing the necessity for frequent or lengthy appointments.

In adult therapy Transforce appliances are comfortable and do not interfere with speech. Arch development is performed efficiently and many irregularities may be treated with invisible appliances throughout treatment by using the lingual approach followed by detailed finishing with Invisalign or lingual brackets. First phase treatment with Transforce appliances would significantly extend the range of malocclusions that may be completed with invisible appliances.

References

Timms D.J. (1968) An occlusal analysis of lateral maxillary expansion with mid palatal suture opening. Trans Eur. Orthod. Soc. Pp 73 – 79

Timms D.J. (1976) Long term follow up of cases treated by rapid maxillary expansion.Trans Eur. Orthod. Soc. Pp 211 - 215.

Melsen B. (1972) A histological study of the influence of sutural morphology and skeletal maturation on rapid palatal expansion in children. Trans Eur. Orthod. Soc. pp 499 - 507

McNamara J.D. & Brudon W.L. (1983) Treatment of tooth-size/ arch-size discrepancy problems. In: orthodontic and orthopedic treatment in the mixed dentition. Needham Press pp 67 -93

Maxillary Transverse Expander

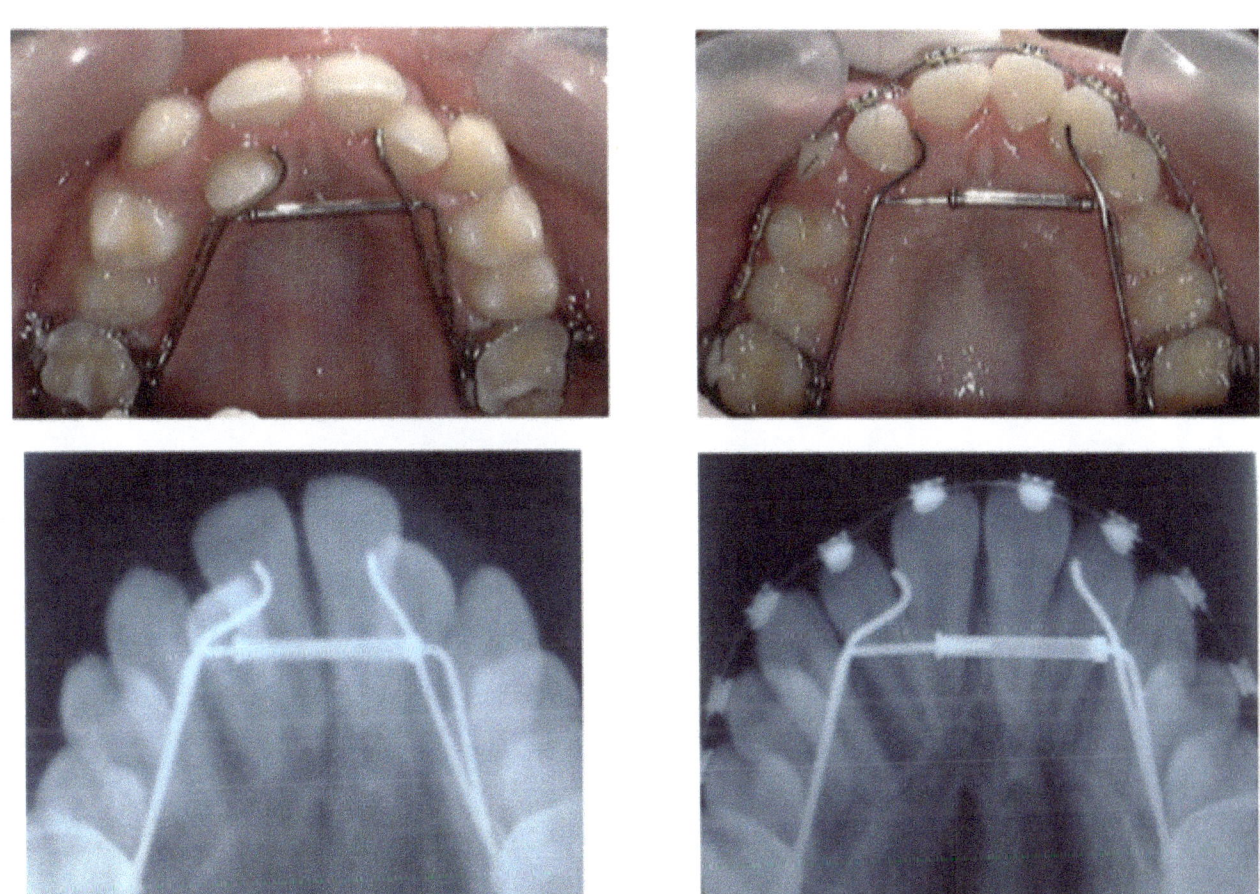

4 months treatment

Mandibular Transverse Expander

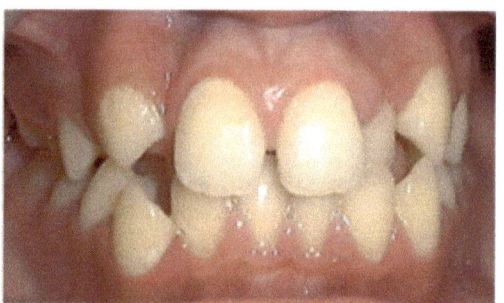

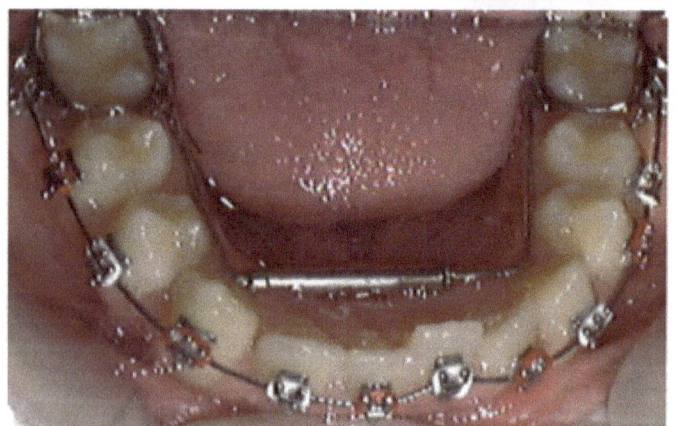
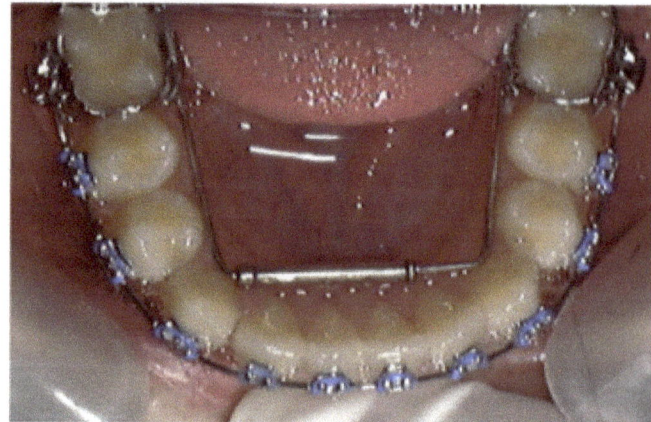

6 months treatment

18 months treatment

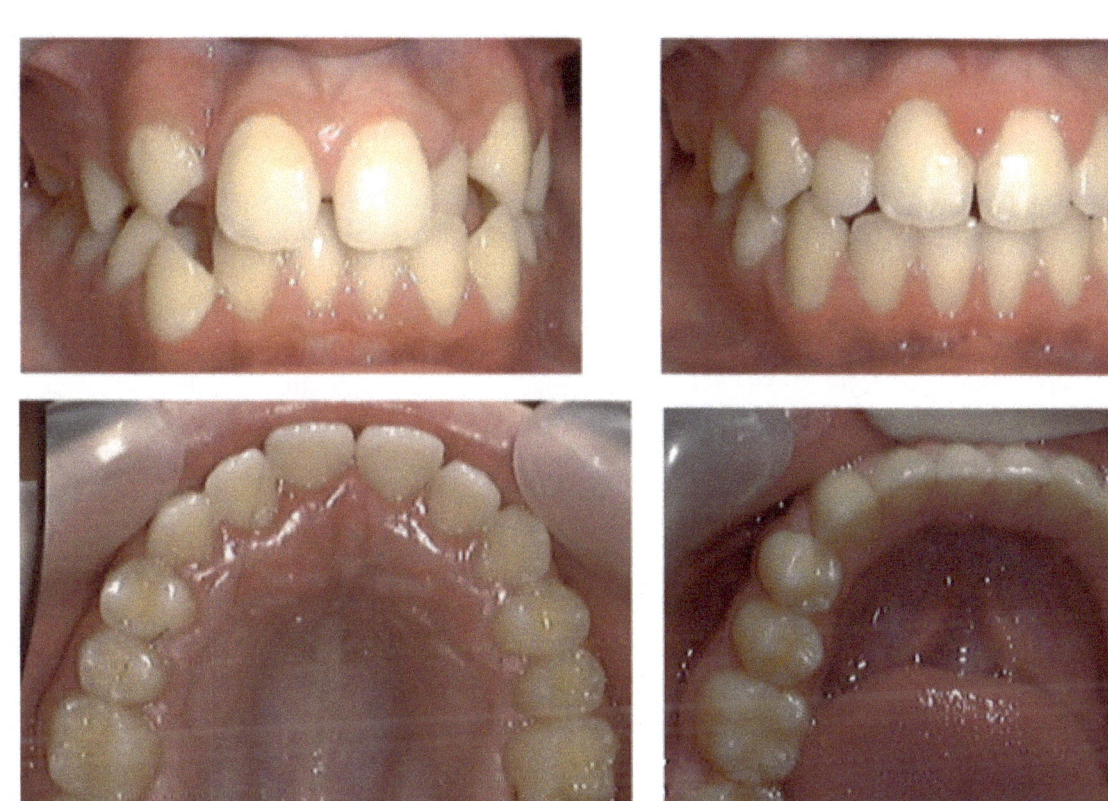

Slow Maxillary Expansion with Nickel Titanium

Roberto Murzban DDS, Ravindra Nanda BDS, MDS, PHD

In animal studies slow expansion procedures have demonstrated orthopaedic effects similar to RPE. Histological examination suggests that sutural separation does occur, but at a rate that maintains the integrity of the maxilllary sutures by allowing for bone remodeling. Clinical studies of human patients in the deciduous or early mixed dentition substantiate these findings. Maxillary width increases ranged from 3.8 mm to 8.7 mm with slow expansion of as much as 1 mm per week using 900 grams of force with the Ni-Ti maxillary expander.

Storey recommends slow expansion at 0.5 to 1 mm per week to allow for "physiological sutural adjustments", which elicit less trauma and a greater repair response compared to rapid maxillary expansion. Ekstrom reports that slowly expanded sutures become well organised in 30 days and are well established with mineralized tissue by three months.

Slow expansion has been found to promote greater post-expansion stability, given an adequate retention period. Furthermore, in comparison of slow expansion with a quad helix and RPE Zachrisson concluded that periodontal breakdown on the buccal aspects of posterior teeth occurred infrequently in both groups, but the few patients who exhibited some attachment loss were in the RPE group.

The Nickel Titanium Expander provides a viable alternative to rapid expansion for correction of transverse discrepancie. Incorporation into an existing fixed appliance eliminates a separate laboratory phase and extra appointments for impressions, adjustments and rebanding molars afer removal. The buccal molar attachments are available for use with intrusion arches, utility arches or comprehensive fixed appliances.

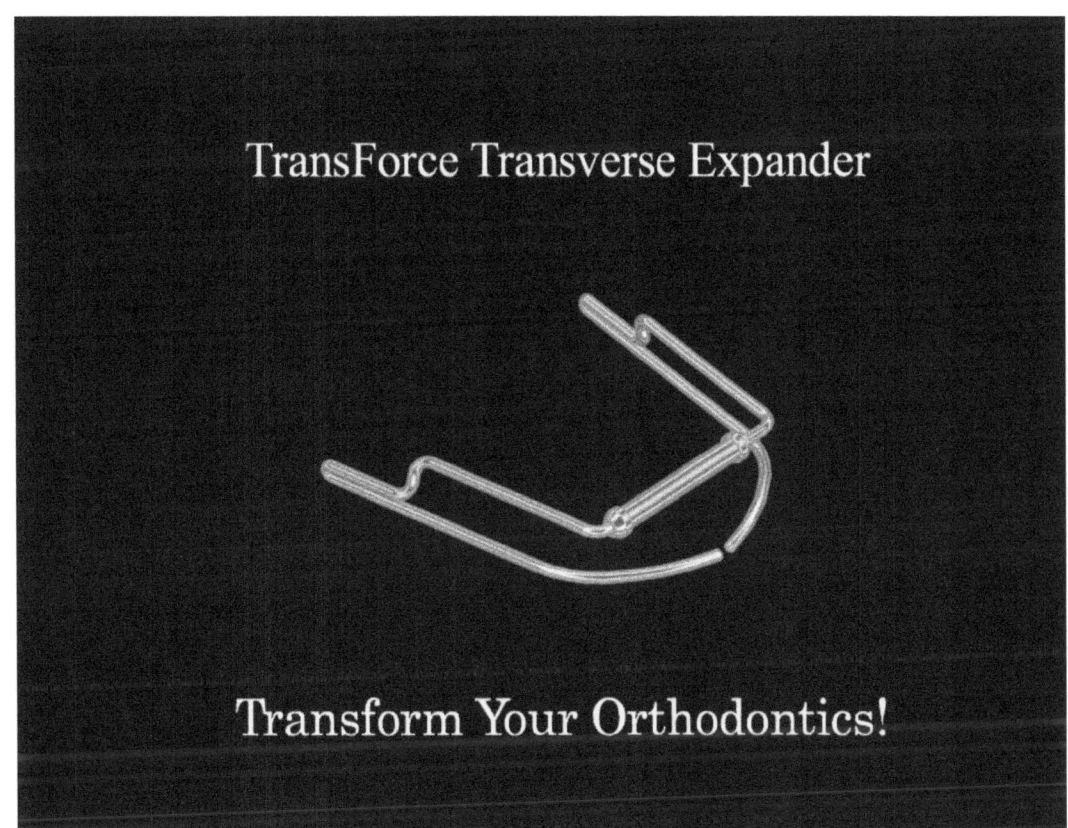

TransForce Transverse Expander

Transform Your Orthodontics!

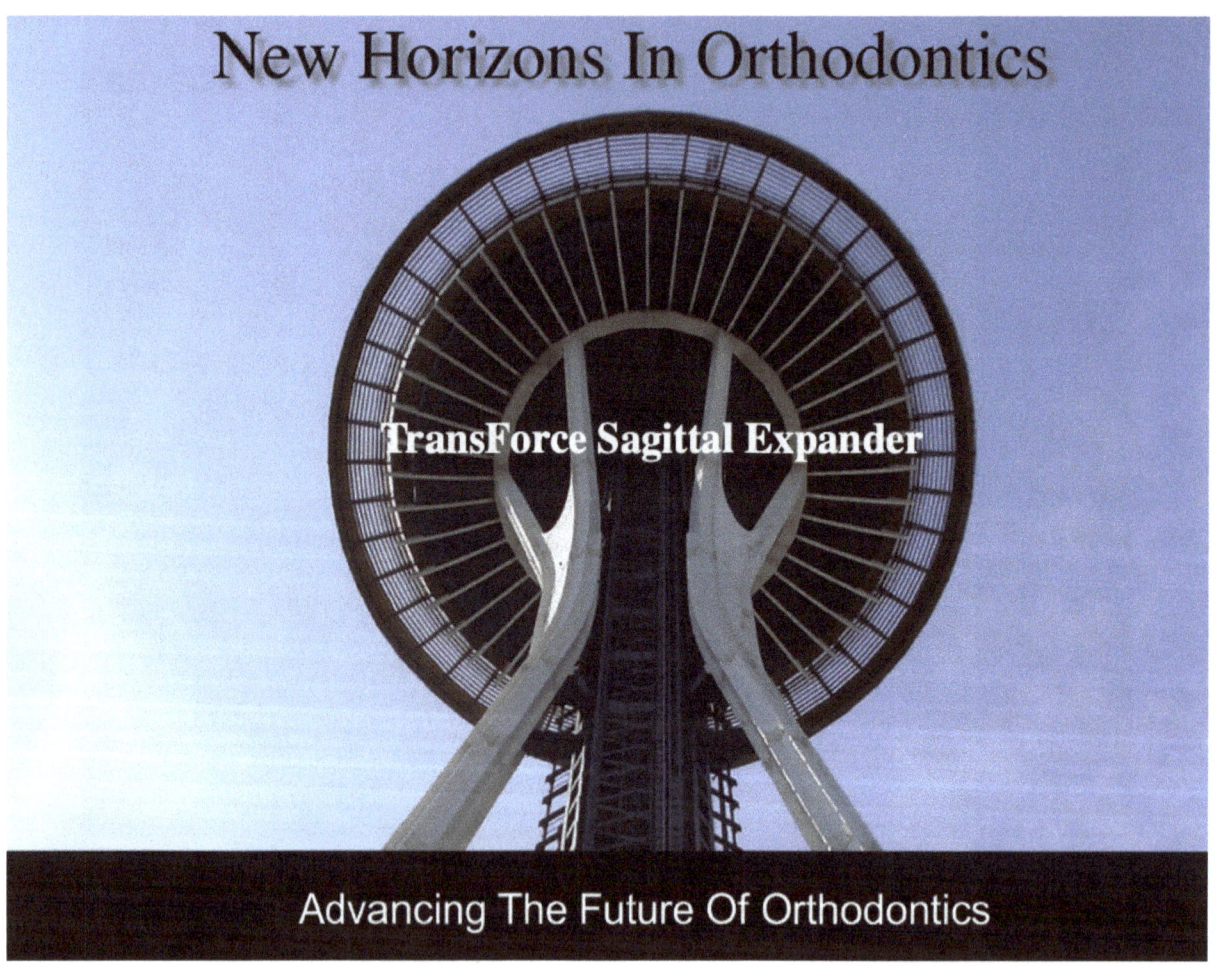

New Horizons In Orthodontics

TransForce Sagittal Expander

Advancing The Future Of Orthodontics

TRANSFORCE 2® SAGITTAL EXPANDER

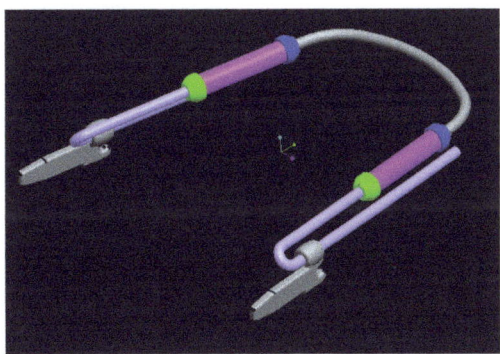

The Sagittal Expander is specifically designed for antero-posterior arch development in upper or lower dental arches, and is often indicated for simultaneous use in both arches.

The sagittal appliance operates on the slide principle and may be used unilaterally or bilaterally to extend arch length. It incorporates bilateral expansion modules, and extends mesially from the molar lingual sheath at gingival level to engage the anterior segment of the dental arch.

In its simplest form the Sagittal Expander applies reciprocal forces between the incisors and molars to lengthen the dental arch and it must be assumed that arch length increase is mainly achieved by incisor proclination unless additional anchorage is used to stabilize the labial segment.

Labial movement of the anterior teeth may be combined with transverse development of the buccal segments where indicated by activating the mesial extension wires to move premolars or deciduous molars, or to expand intercanine width. As the modules expand this also achieves expansion of the inter-molar width. The sagittal appliance is pre-activated to achieve the amount of expansion required.

Custom modification for distal movement of molars is possible by cutting the anterior wire in the midline and bending the wires into the palate to be incorporated in a Nance button. Anterior anchorage may be reinforced to achieve this objective during fixed appliance therapy or alternatively implants may be used to achieve additional stationary anchorage.

The Sagittal Expander is provided in seven sizes. The mesio-distal length of the appliances varies by 2 mm increments throughout the range. The range of action of the sagittal appliance is 6 mm in the larger sizes, which are used only in the upper arch. The smaller sizes with 4 mm range of action, can be used in the upper or lower arch. Careful selection is advised to provide the correct amount of tooth movement required for each individual case.

Both Sagittal and Transverse appliances have additional components to achieve 3-way expansion where this is indicated. The invisible lingual appliances may be used in correction of all classes of malocclusion at any stage of development from mixed dentition through permanent dentition and this approach has wide indications in adult treatment.

Transforce lingual appliances are readily integrated with conventional fixed appliances. In addition arch development with lingual appliances may be combined with lingual brackets or invisable appliances to complete treatment. The lingual approach has excellent potential in adult treatment, especially as the appliances do not cover the palate and do not interfere with speech.

Sagittal Arch Development

Guidelines For Case Selection

Sagittal Arch Development is required when arch length is constricted by retroclined upper or lower incisors, as commonly found in Class II Division 2 malocclusion and Class I malocclusion with bimaxillary retrusion. These patients generally present with deep overbite and reduced lower facial height, and whenever possible should be treated without extractions to maintain or improve the vertical dimension. Sagittal arch development helps to resolve anterior crowding, and proclination of the incisors reduces the overbite.

Sagittal correction is by labial movement of anterior teeth, and may be accompanied by slight distal movement and disto-lingual rotation of molars.

It is essential to confirm that adequate bony support is available before proclining incisors, and it is especially important not to procline incisors that are already procumbent or are correctly related to the mandibular base. An essential objective in treatment planning is to place the lower incisors in a stable position over basal bone. The protocol in diagnosis should therefore be determined by arch length analysis from study models and cephalometric analysis to determine upper and lower incisor position for correct case selection.

Labial movement of lower incisors is only indicated if they are retroclined and the tip of the incisor is positioned significantly lingual to the A/Po line. Ideally for aesthetic and functional balance, the lower incisors should be positioned in the range of 1 to 3 mm ahead of the A-Po line at the end of treatment.

When a lateral incisor is displaced lingual to a central incisor, it is advisable to expand the arch transversely before advancing the lateral incisor, in order to avoid moving the central incisor labially out of the alveolar trough.

Dental Class III malocclusion with retroclined upper incisors is generally suitable for sagittal arch development by proclination of upper incisors. Many such malocclusions also benefit from transverse expansion and ideally should be treated in mixed dentition. To differentiate from a true skeletal Class III pattern the patient should be able to meet the incisors edge to edge before posturing forward to entrap the upper incisors in lingual occlusion.

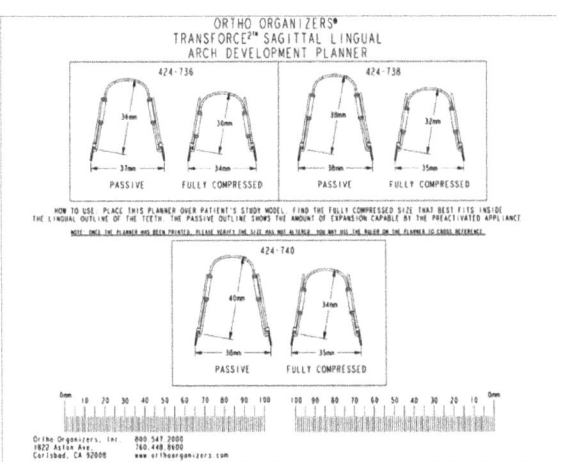

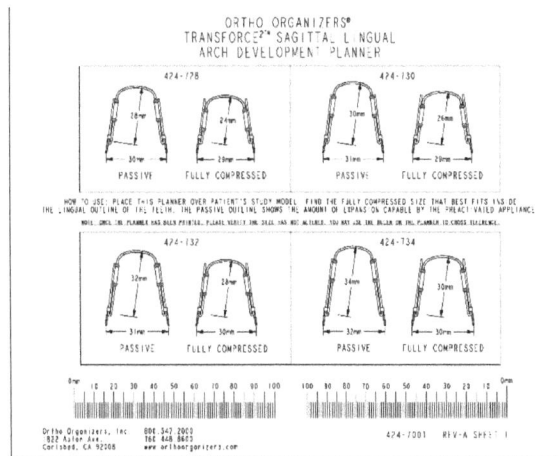

A clear template is provided by Ortho Organizers showing a scale model of the appliance in both compressed and fully extended forms. The template is placed over the occlusal surface of a model to measure arch length and molar width.

The template provides a visual guide to facilitate selection of the appropriate size of the appliance. The size is selected to fit the individual patient by laying the template over a study model. The compressed outline of the appliance should fit inside the lingual outline of the teeth. The extended outline shows the amount of pre-activation in the appliance.

Alternatively the millimetre scale on the template may be used to measure arch length on the model before treatment. The length on each side of the arch is measured from the molar point (level with the mesio-lingual cusp) to the incisal point (the gingival papilla between the central incisors). This distance may be compared with the compressed length of the Sagitttal Expander on the template from the mesial edge of the lingual sheath to the mid point of the anterior section. The extended image of the appliance on the template is a guide to the number of millimetres activation present in the coil springs.

Before fitting the appliance it is useful to check the range of activation by placing the assembled appliance on the model. The bands fit over the molars and the lingual arch is engaged on the incisors to observe the range of action when the coil springs are compressed.

The larger sizes have 6 mm range of activation and are only suitable for the upper arch. The smaller sizes have 4 mm activation and can also be used selectively in the lower arch.

Selecting the Correct Size of TransForce Sagittal Expander

A clear template is provided by Ortho Organizers showing a scale model of the appliance in both compressed and fully extended forms. The template is placed over the occlusal surface of a model to measure arch length and molar width.

The template provides a visual guide to facilitate selection of the appropriate size of the appliance. The compressed outline of the appliance should fit inside the lingual outline of the teeth. The extended outline shows the amount of pre-activation in the appliance.

Before fitting the appliance it is useful to check the range of activation by placing the assembled appliance on the model. The bands fit over the molars and the lingual arch is engaged on the incisors to observe the range of action when the coil springs are compressed.

The larger sizes have 6 mm range of activation and are only suitable for the upper arch. The smaller sizes have 4 mm activation and can also be used selectively in the lower arch

The template displays an outline of the appliance in the fully compressed and fully extended size. The correct size is selected by overlaying the image of the appliance

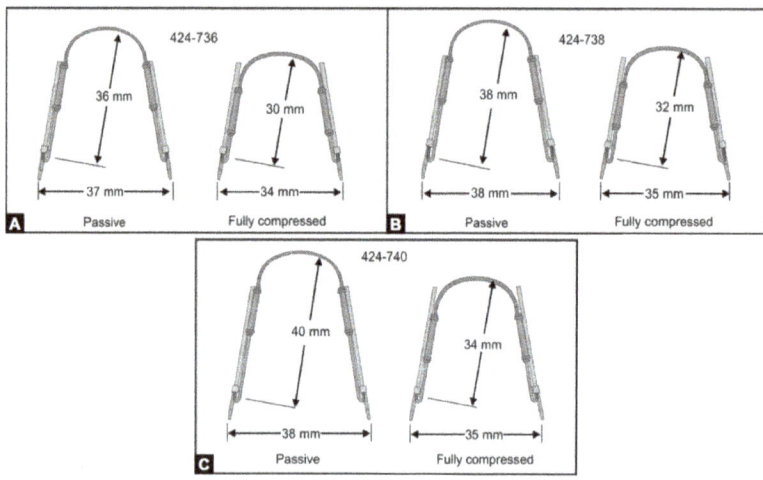

on the model. If required the anterior extension wires can be adapted to act on individual teeth. Overlaying the passive image will predict the amount of expansion that will be delivered by the appliance as the compression units expand   The smaller sizes have a range of action of 4 mm from fully compressed to fully extended. They may be used in the upper or lower arch. They are more likely to be fully compressed in the upper arch. This would accommodate up to 8 mm of crowding in the buccal segments by advancing the upper incisors. When less crowding is present, the next smaller size of sagittal appliance will accommodate up to 4 mm of crowding from fully compressed to fully extended.

Case selection is important, and the sagittal appliance should be used only in the lower arch when proclination of the lower incisors is indicated, e.g. when the lower incisors are retroclined and positioned lingual to the A-pogonion line.

In planning treatment, calculate the number of mm of crowding, the Arch Length Discrepancy (ALD), and divide by 2. Each mm of advancement of the lower incisors will accommodate 2 mm of crowding. This gives an estimate of the final position of the lower incisors relative to the A-pogonion line.

The ideal position of the tip of the lower incisor after treatment is in the range of +1 to +3 mm to the A-pogonion line. The limit of +3 mm may apply to brachyfacial faces. In mesofacial faces +1 mm may be the ideal position. Sagittal advancement of the lower incisor is seldom indicated in dolichofacial faces with long, thin alveolar processes due to a lack of bony support. The sagittal appliance is then contraindicated.

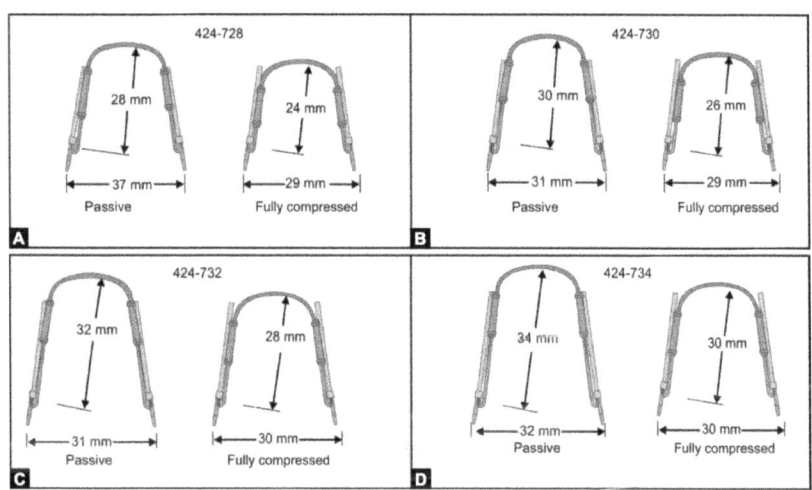

Using the Sagittal Template

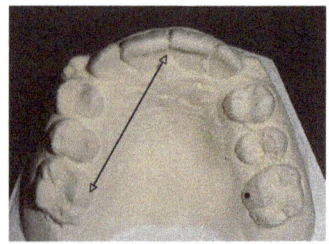

Measure Sagittal Length

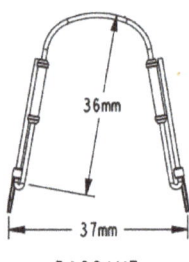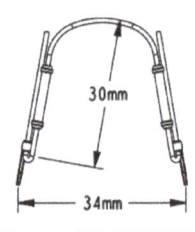

PASSIVE   FULLY COMPRESSED

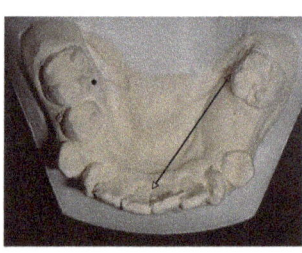

Measure Sagittal Length

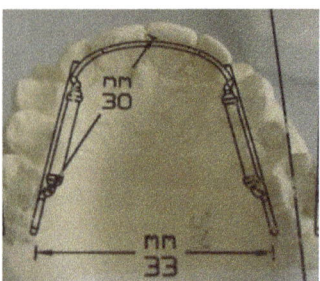

Upper Before & After

The template displays an outline of the appliance in the fully compressed and fully extended size. An estimate of the size can be obtained by measuring the sagittal length on the model. The correct size is selected by overlaying the image of the appliance on the model. The compressed image must fit inside the arch before treatment. If required the anterior extension wires can be adapted to act on individual teeth. Overlaying the passive image will predict the amount of expansion that will be delivered by the appliance as the compression unit expands.

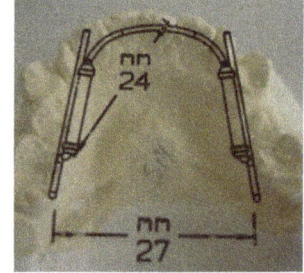

Lower Before & After

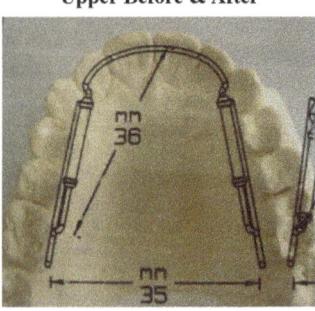

This patient was treated by arch development in early permanent dentition and the images show the amount of arch development. The upper models before and after treatment are on the left and the lower models on the right.

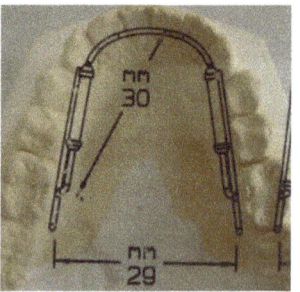

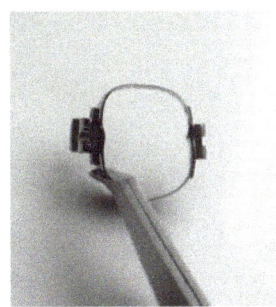

Horizontal Lingual Sheath

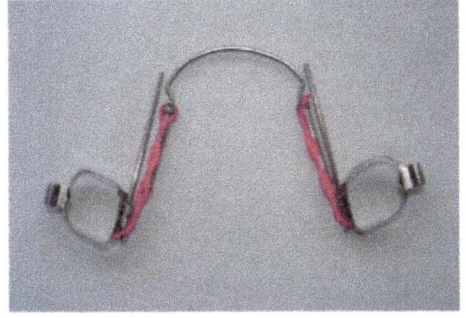

Fitting TransForce Sagittal Appliances

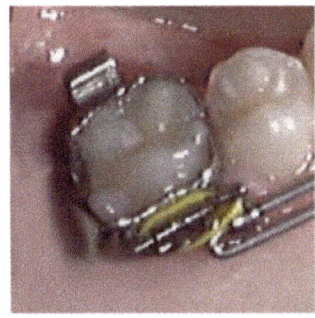

Elastic Tie-back

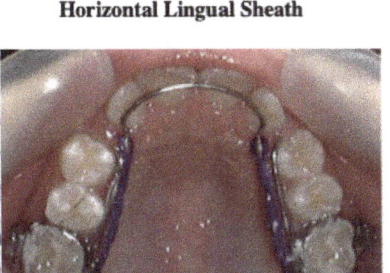

Composite added

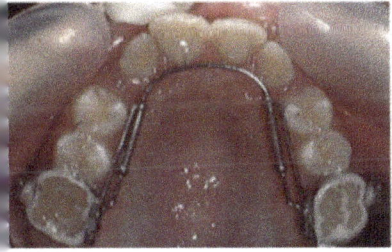

Separators must be placed, preferably within 3 days of the appointment to fit the appliance. Molar bands with horizontal lingual sheaths are selected and the appliance is fully assembled and tried in the mouth prior to cementing. Minor adjustment may be required to adapt the appliance to the individual patient. If required a lingual button or composite can be added to engage the wire correctly on upper incisors.

The appliance may be prepared on models using an Essix delivery tray to fit by an indirect technique. This makes it easier to fit the appliance when the springs are fully compressed.

For a direct technique one band is placed before engaging the wire lingual to the incisors. Compress the spring on the other side against the resistance of the incisors to fit the band on the other side. An elastic chain module may sometimes be used to compress the appliance

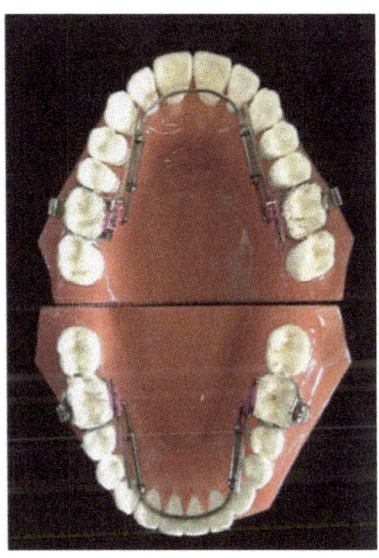

Maintenance & Adjustment

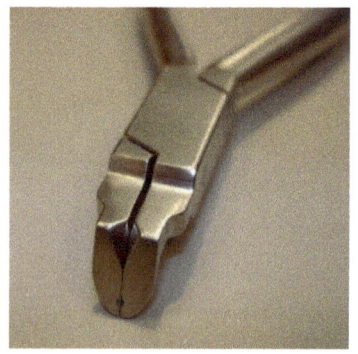 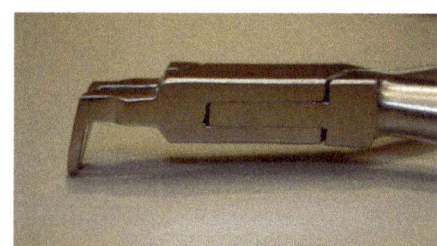 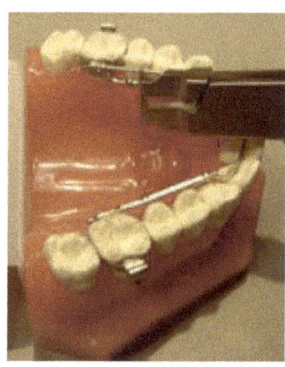

Maintenance is minimal and may be limited to routine visits at 6 to 8 week intervals to check progress. The mesial extension wires on the sagittal appliance may be adjusted intra-orally with triple beak or concavo-convex pliers to control expansion of the premolars and canines.

At any stage in treatment crimping pliers may be used to compress the tube on the wire close to the distal end stop of the expansion module on the sagittal appliance to make the appliance passive and prevent further activation. Angled crimping pliers have been developed by Ortho Organizers for this purpose.

It is preferable to select the size of appliance carefully to deliver the amount of sagittal activation required to advance the incisors, rather than select a size that is too large and requires to be de-activated

In transverse arch development it is essential to expand the inter-canine width to accommodate lingually displaced incisors before activating to advance the incisors. The lingual wires should remain passive until space has been created to accommodate the instanding incisors. Intra-oral adjustment of the labial extensions on the transverse appliance may then control the alignment of the incisors.

ARCH DEVELOPMENT PLANNING

This boy has a Class I buccal segment relationship with retroclined upper central incisors and crowding of the lower labial segment. Upper and lower TransForce Sagittal appliances were used to correct archform and align the anterior teeth. The lower appliance was fitted first to advance the lower incisors and reduce the overbite before fitting the upper sagittal appliance. This avoids having the lower incisors damaging the upper appliance in deep overbite cases.

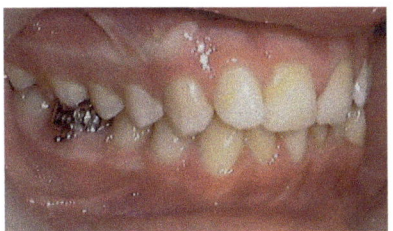 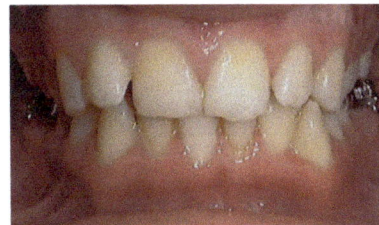 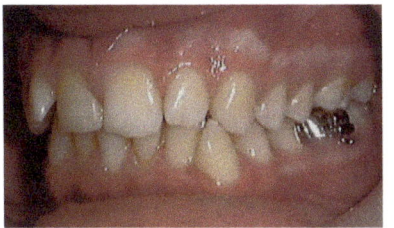

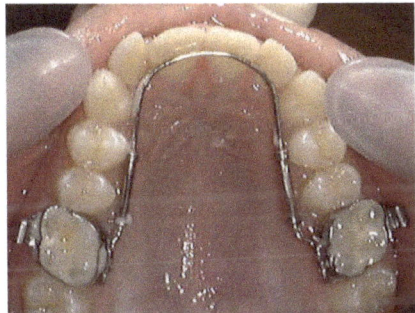 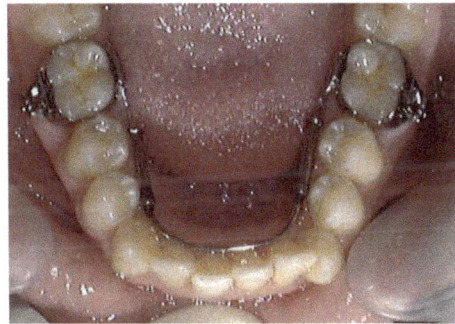

SIMULATED ARCH DEVELOPMENT

Arch development can be planned on computer by digitizing the models to show the position and size of the teeth on an occlusogram. The computer programme can evaluate the crowding present and the A-Pogoinion line can be assessed on the cephalogram and transferred to the occlusogram to visualize the position of the anterior teeth. The treatment is planned by moving the teeth to correct the alignment on computer and checking their relationship to the A-Pogonion line to evaluate the stability of the end result before fitting the appliances

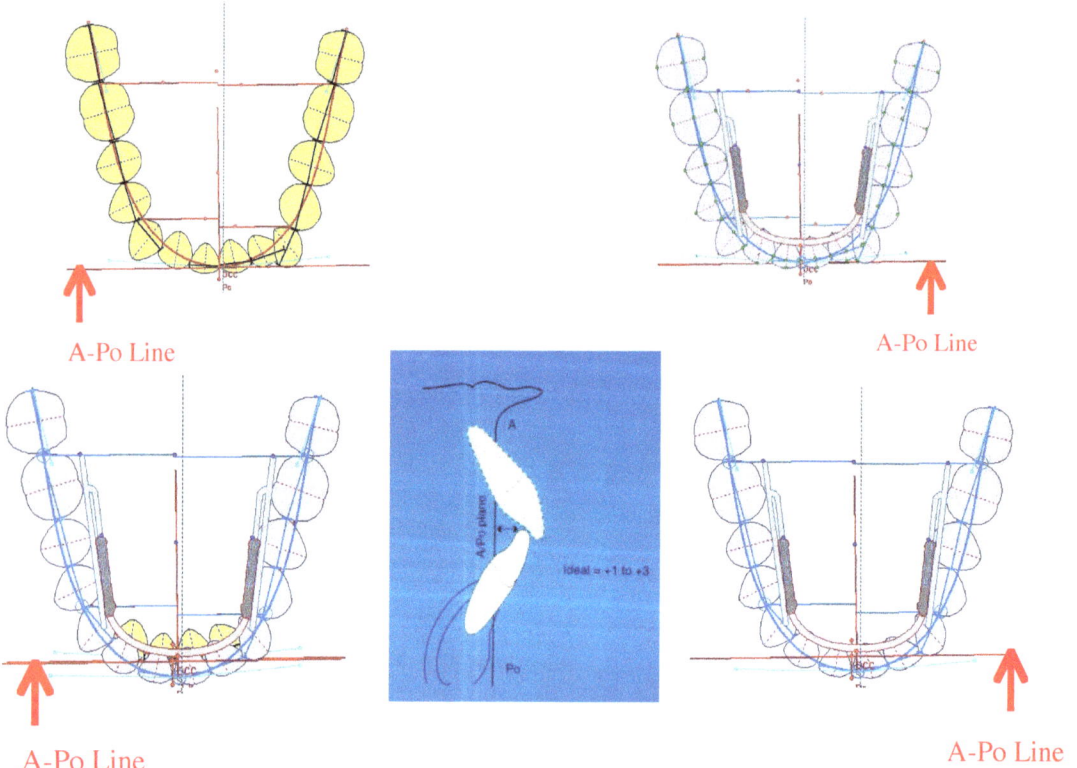

A-Po Line

A-Po Line

A-Po Line

A-Po Line

SIMULATED ARCH DEVELOPMENT

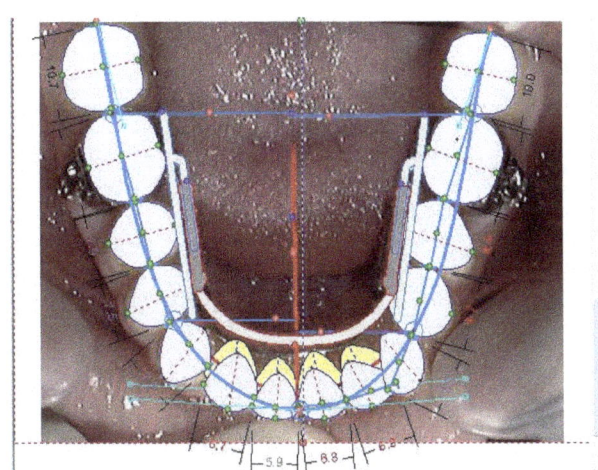

Tramo???	Long. Av	Long Nec	Discrep.
Of 12 to 22			
Of 15 to 25			
Of 16 to 26			
Of 17 to 18,			
Of 18 to 28			
ADI	**Right**		
Tramo???	Long. Av	Long Nec	Discrep.
Of 41 to 42	12.72	12.66	0.06
Of 41 to 45	36.08	35.28	0.80
Of 41 to 46	47.65	46.51	1.14
Of 47 to 48	11.51	10.67	0.84
Of 41 to 48	59.16	57.18	1.98
ADI	**Left**		
Tramo???	Long. Av	Long Nec	Discrep.
Of 31 to 32	11.84	13.19	-1.35
Of 31 to 35	35.54	37.55	-2.01
Of 31 to 36	46.75	48.55	-1.80
Of 37 to 38	10.69	10.02	0.67
Of 31 to 38	57.44	58.57	-1.13
ADI	**Total**		
Tramo???	Long. Av	Long Nec	Discrep.
Of 32 to 42	24.56	25.85	-1.29
Of 35 to 45	71.62	72.83	-1.21
Of 36 to 46	94.40	95.06	-0.66

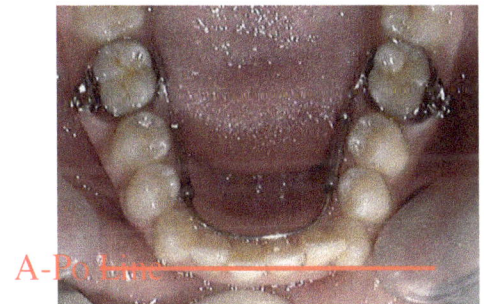

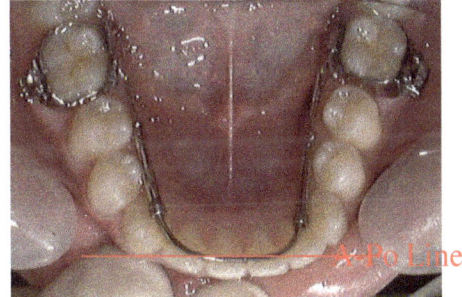

This shows the improvement in arch form after 9 months treatment

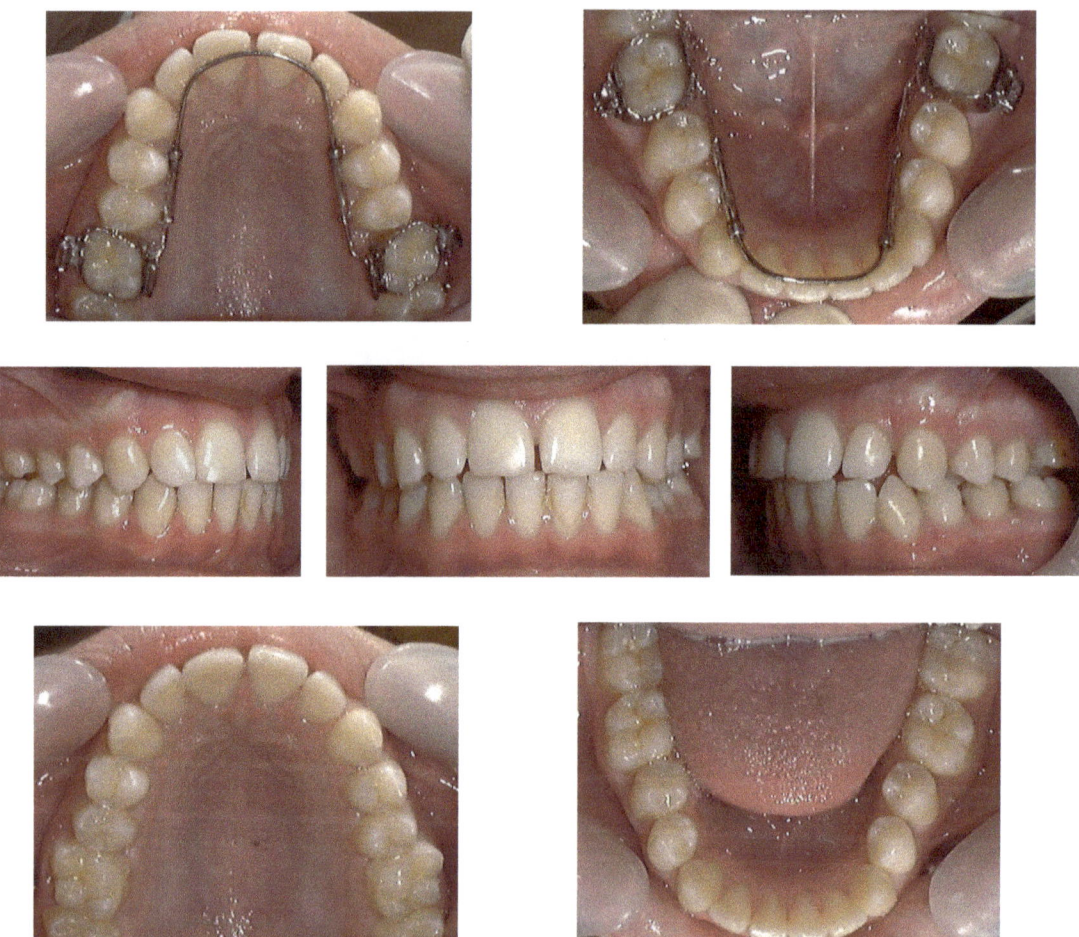

OPTIONS FOR FINISHING TREATMENT

Correction of alignment with invisible lingual appliances is free of friction and occurs more rapidly than other types of aesthetic or invisible appliances. This approach is less expensive and more comfortable than alternative appliances. At this stage there are options on how to finish treatment and retain the position. If required detailing can be carried out by labial or lingual fixed appliances, or alternatively by invisible appliances. This approach is a very attractive option in adult treatment and can be followed by fixed lingual retainers to complete treatment with invisIble appliances

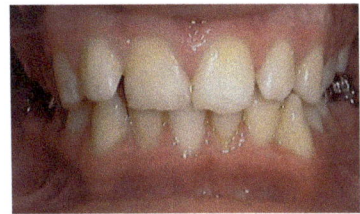 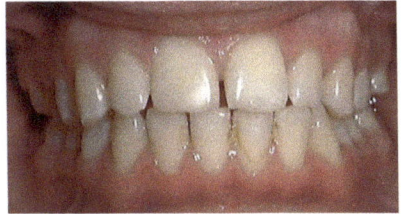 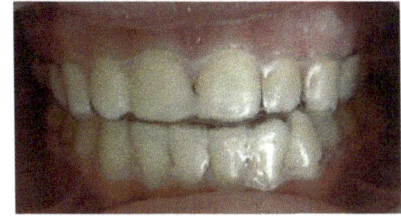

13 Years 6 Months   16 Years 1 Month

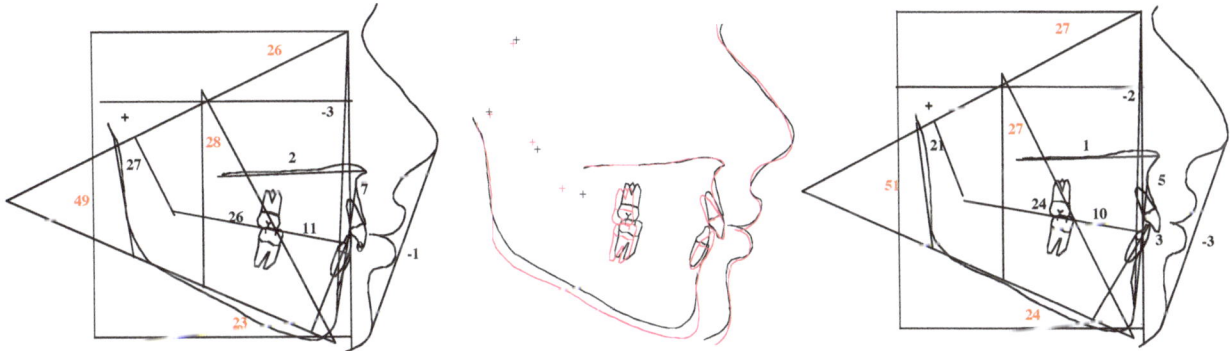

Treated with Invisible TransForce Appliances

This correction was achieved with invisible lingual appliances without fixed appliances. Rapid tooth movements occur without any frictional resistance. This concept can be used from mixed dentition to adult dentition. In adult therapy invisible appliances may be used for detailed finishing and fixed lingual retainers can be fitted for long-term retention

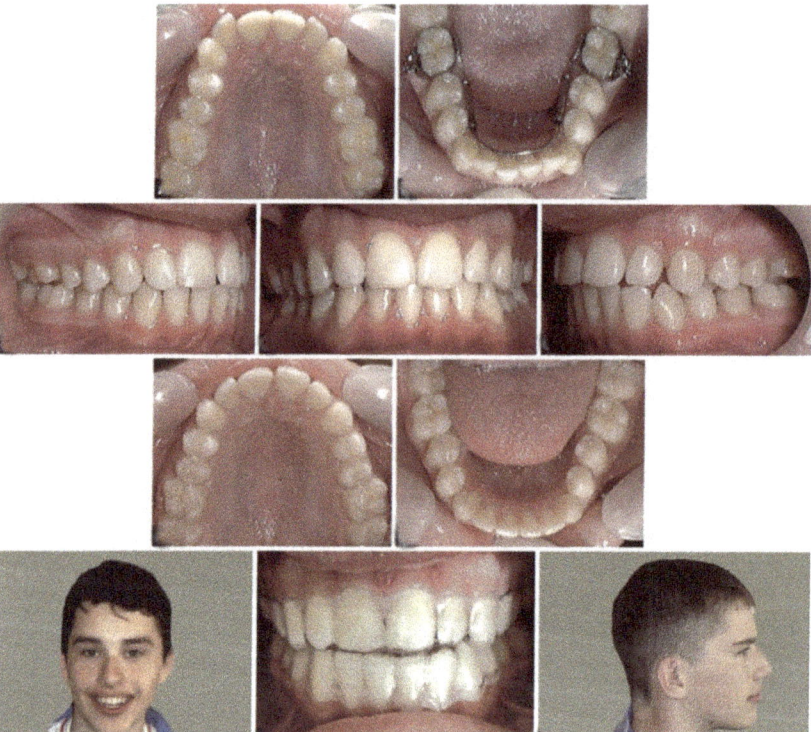

SAGITTAL DEVELOPMENT IN CLASS III MALOCCLUSION

This case illustrates Interceptive treatment for a Class III malocclusion in mixed dentition with an upper Sagittal *Transforce* appliance. The lingual occlusion was corrected after 3 months, and the appliance was used as a retainer for a further 6 months.

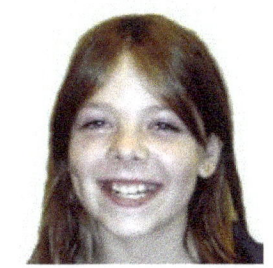
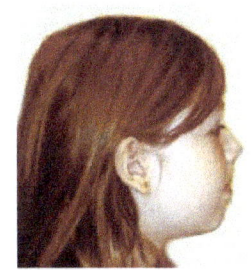

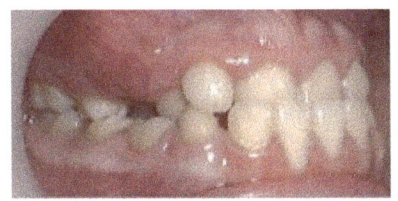
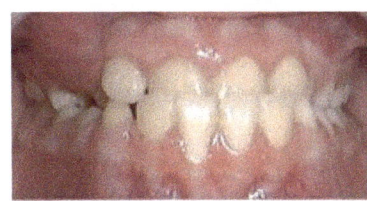
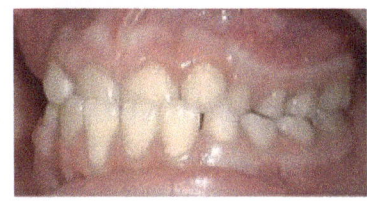

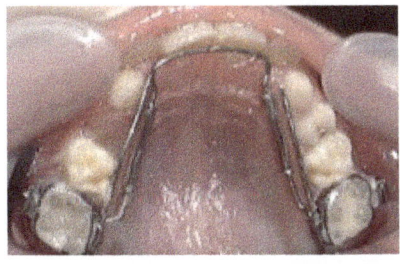
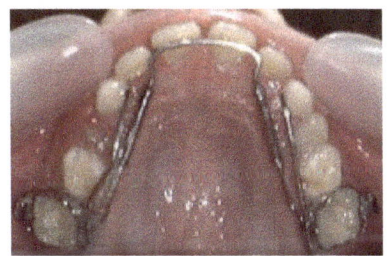

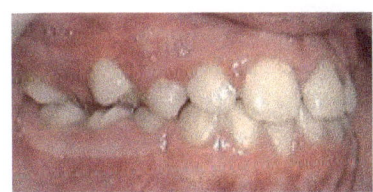
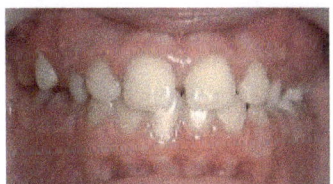
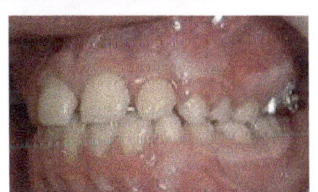

Cranial Base Angle 28°: Facial Axis 24°: Mandibular Plane 25° Convexity 2 mm

A Class I skeletal pattern with 2 mm convexity indicates that only orthodontic correction is required. Upper incisors are retroclined and lower incisors proclined with the incisal edges 8 mm labial to the line from A to Pogonion. The maxillary response to sagittal development is favourable and produces an improvement in the profile

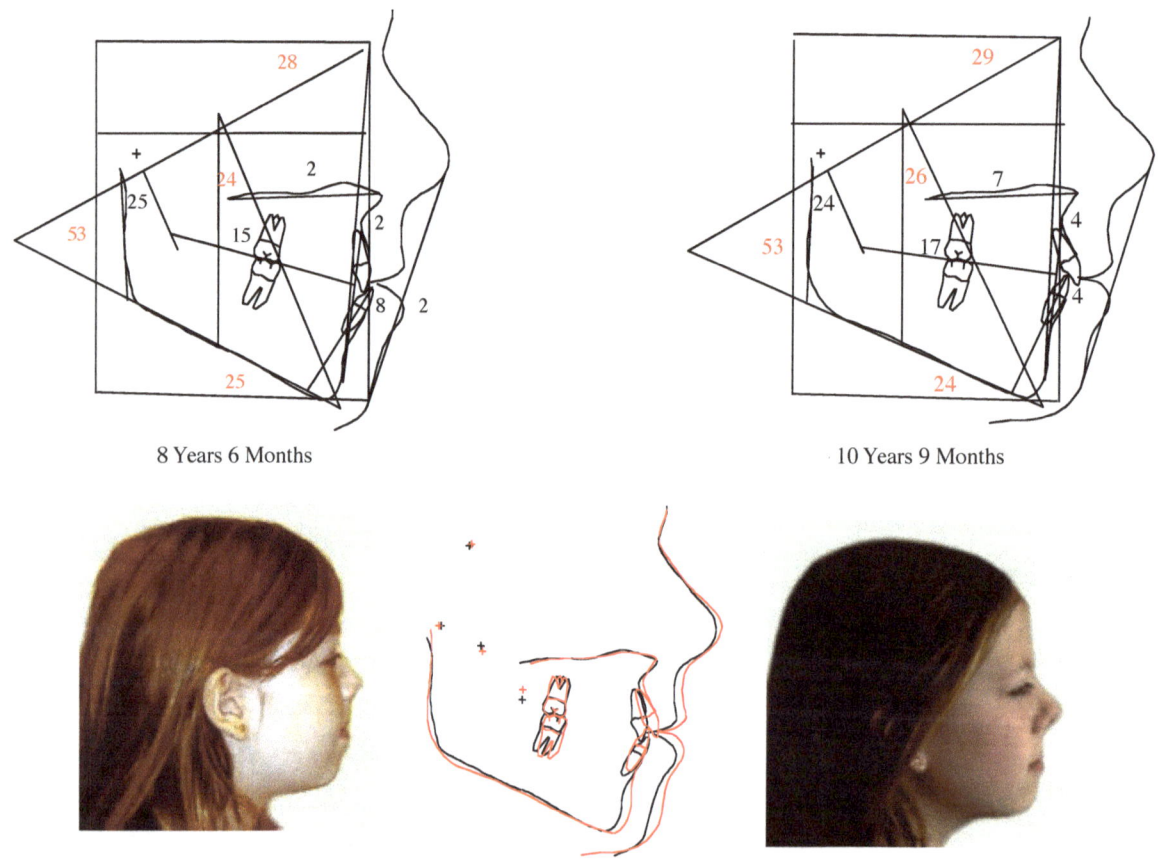

8 Years 6 Months   10 Years 9 Months

No further treatment was required and the final photographs show the occlusion and arch form three years later after eruption of permanent teeth. The profile and facial balance has improved after a short period of interceptive treatment with a Sagittal *Transforce* appliance.

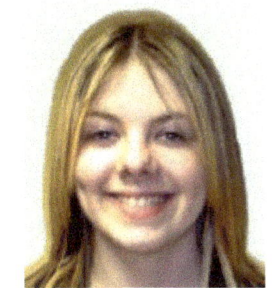
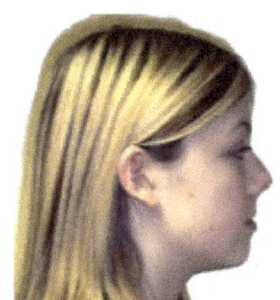

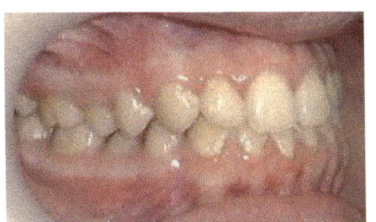
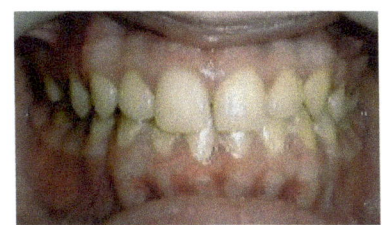
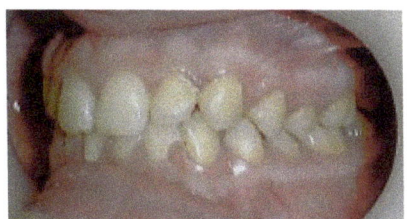

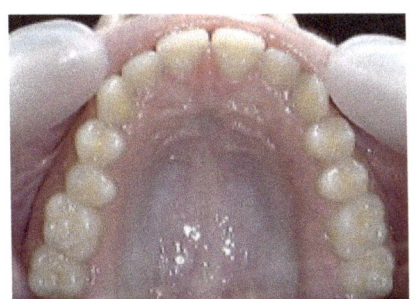
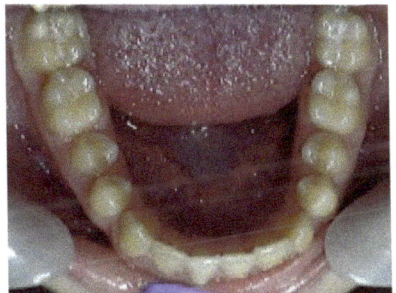

POSTURAL MANDIBULAR DISPLACEMENT

An example of simple treatment to correct a postural mandibiular displacement in a mild Class III malocclusion using a TransForce Sagittal appliance to align the anterior teeth and simultaneously widen the upper arch. Before treatment the mandible is displaced to the left in occlusion

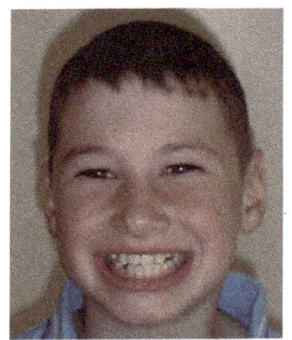
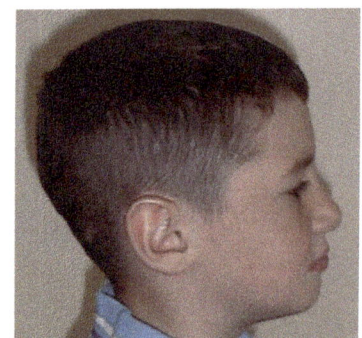

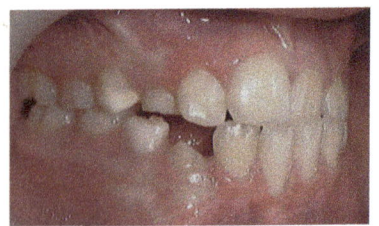
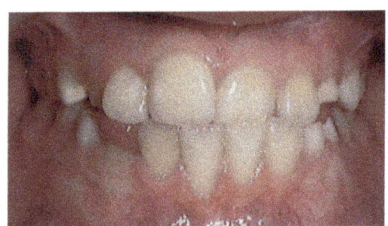
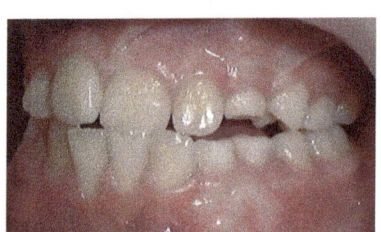

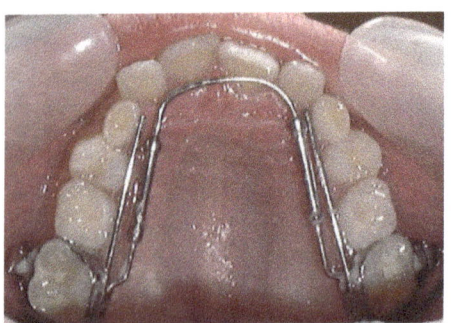
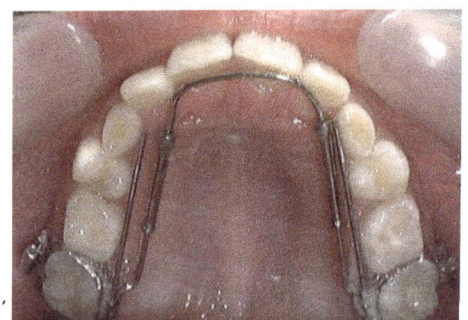

Treatment was completed in 4 months, when the mandibular displacement has improved. One year out of retention the premolars and canines had erupted and no further treatment was required.

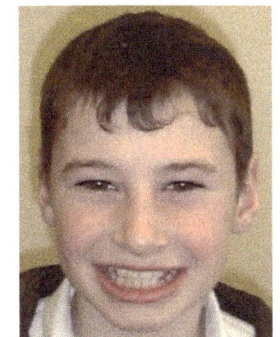
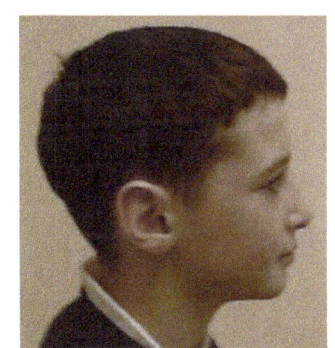

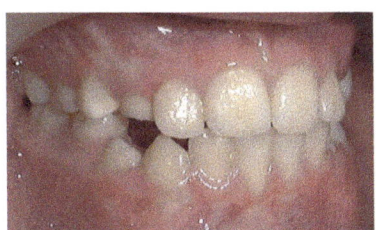
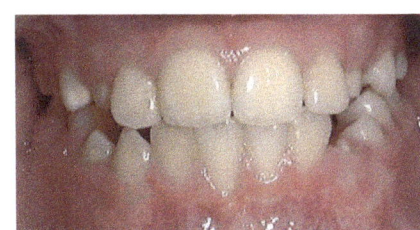
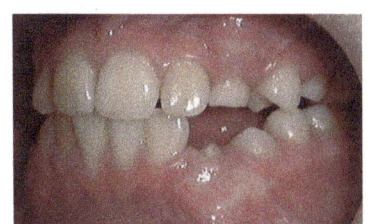

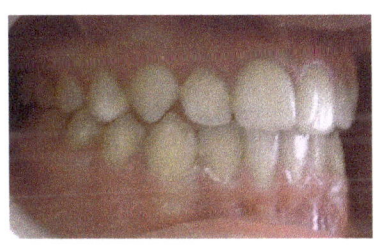
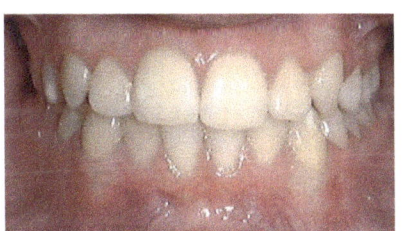
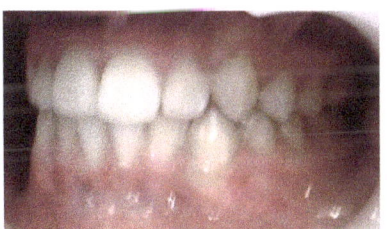

Final records show the position 4 years after treatment. The occlusion is stable, and
the Class III growth pattern is still evident

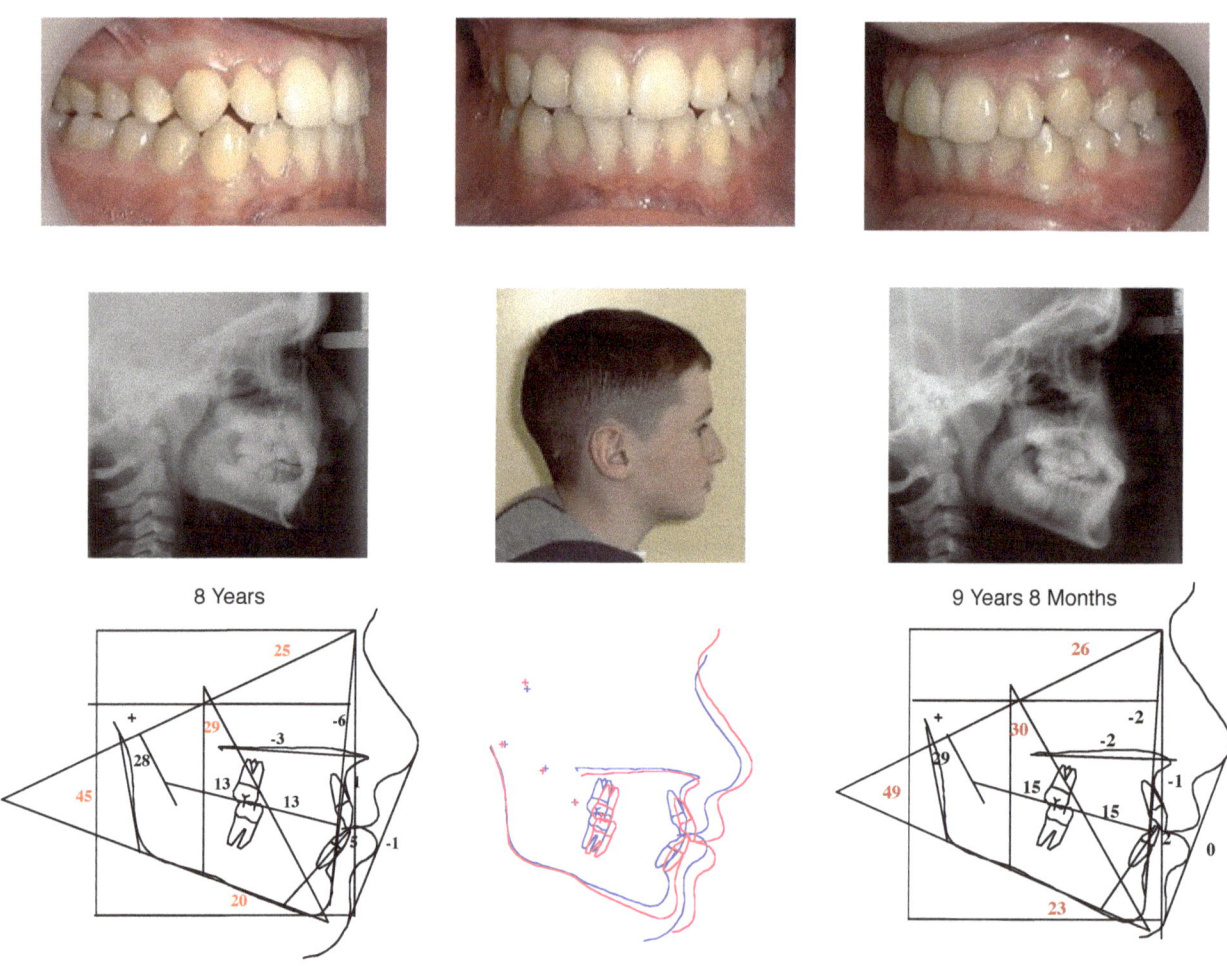

8 Years

9 Years 8 Months

MILD CLASS III MALOCCLUSION IN TRANSITIONAL DENTITION

This 10 year old presents a malocclusion with a Class III growth pattern in mixed dentition. Interceptive treatment is required for crowding and lingual occlusion of the upper central incisors at this stage. Treatment would aim to correct the malocclusion, align the upper incisors and improve arch form to accommodate the unerupted upper canines. There is mild lower labial crowding and slight gingival recession of 1/1 related to the traumatic occlusion of the incisors.

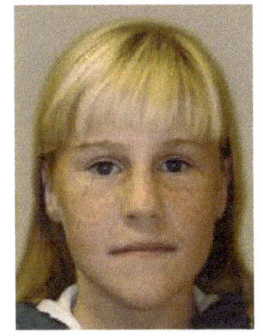 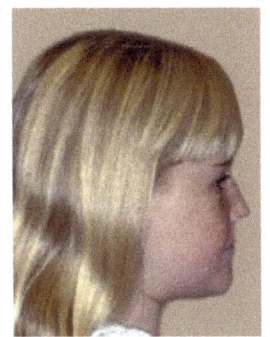

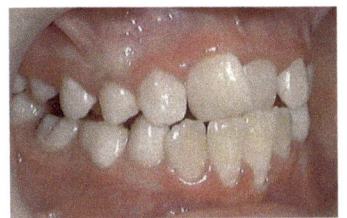 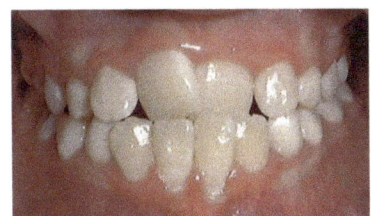 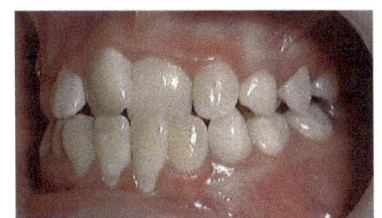

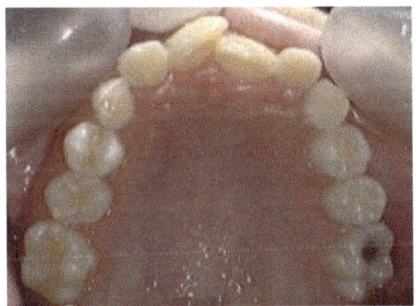 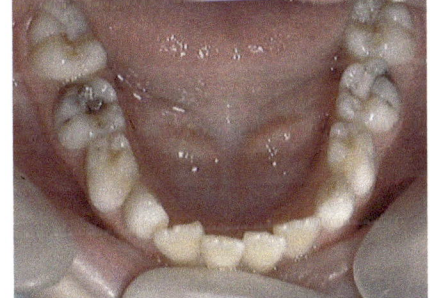

A Sagittal Transforce appliance is fitted first to advance the central incisors and correct the lingual occlusion. This is followed by a simple fixed appliance to improve alignment and to make space to accommodate the upper canines. This phase of treatment was completed in one year, and appliances were removed, waiting eruption of canines.

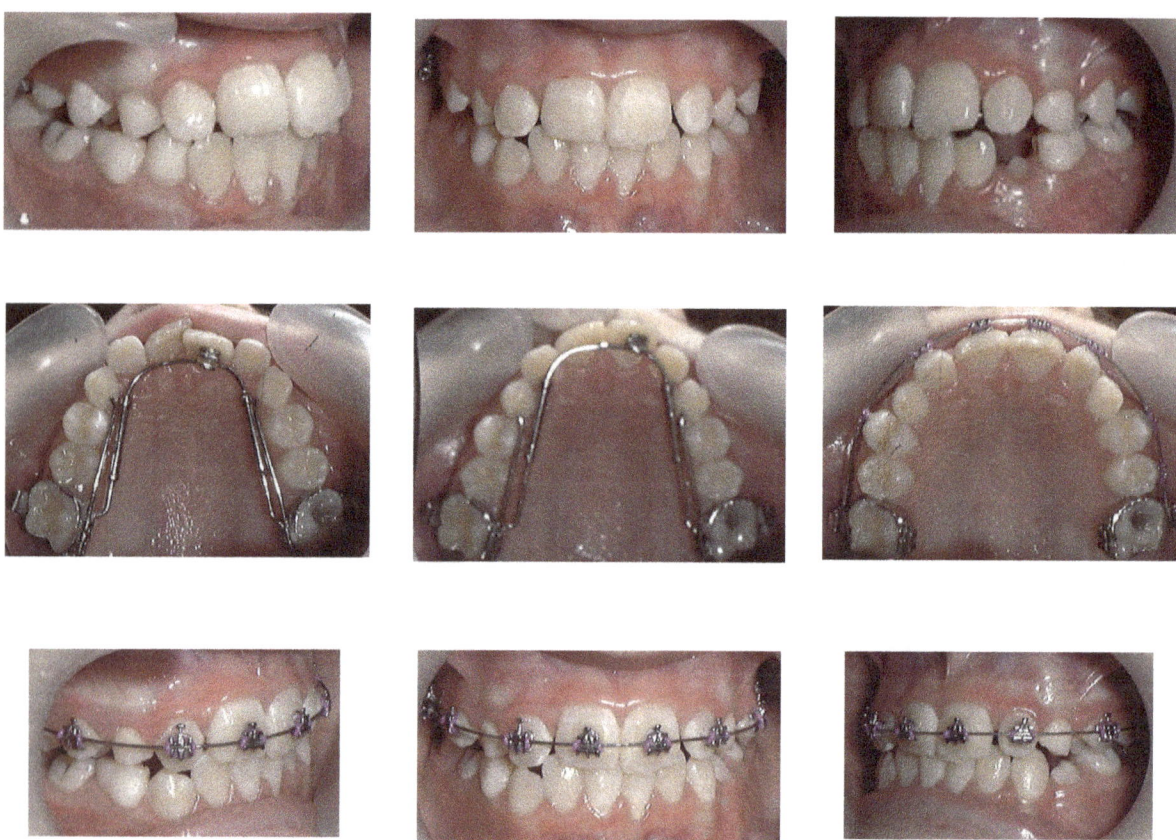

A period of observation followed before resuming treatment at age 14 with upper and lower fixed appliances to detail the occlusion. Delta Force brackets are used as the 22° torque in the upper incisors is an advantage in this Class III pattern.

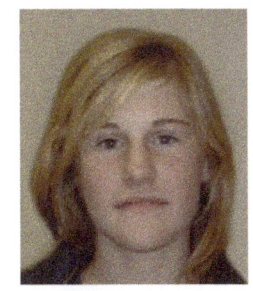
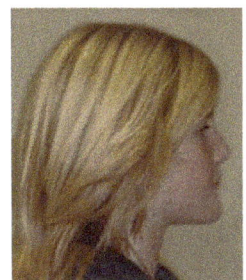

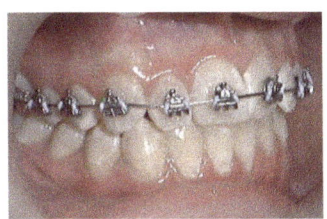
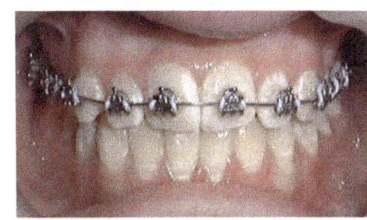
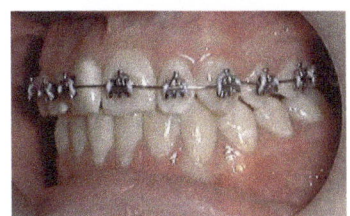

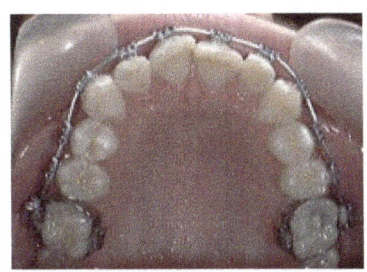
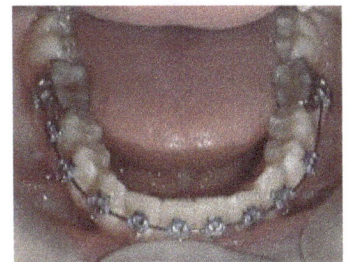

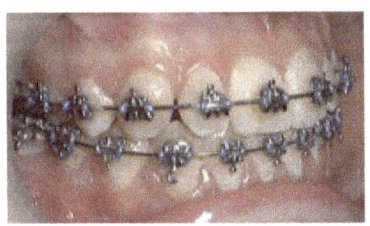
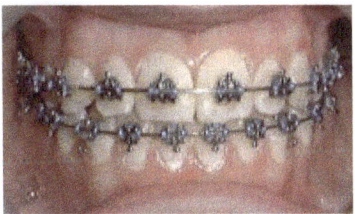
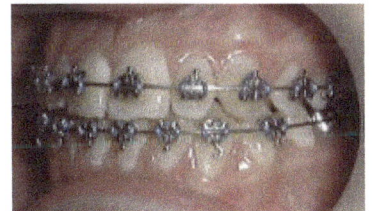

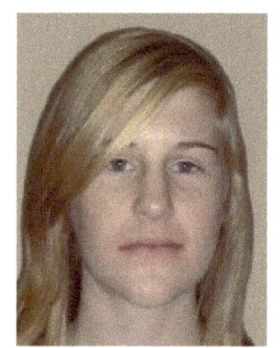
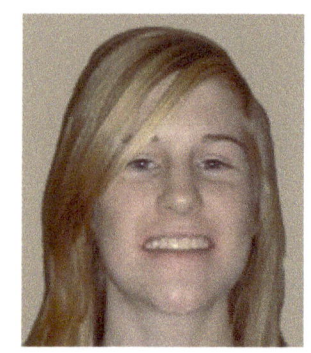
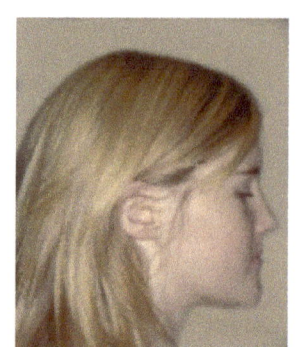
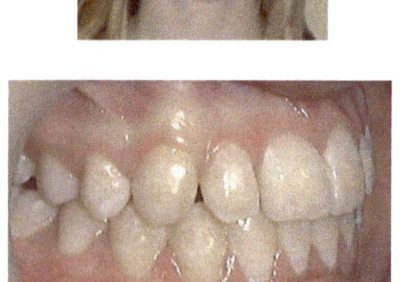
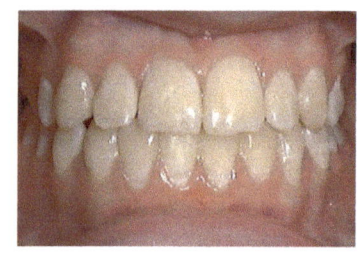
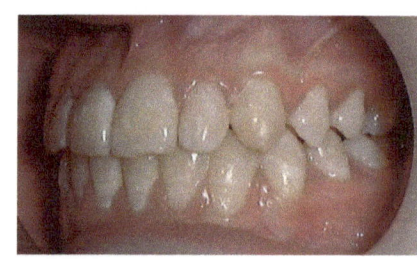
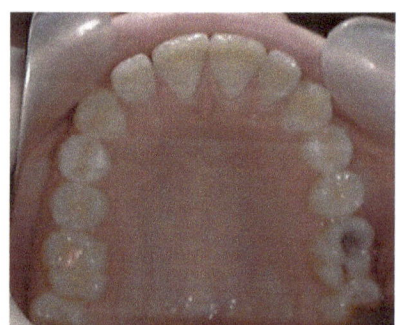
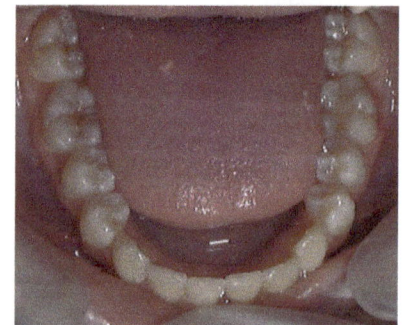

Retention in this case was by removable retainers, which still provide a valid alternative to fixed lingual retainers. After a period of full time retention they can be reduced to night time wear and continue to be monitored as required. The patient is instructed to return for review if the appliances feel tight when inserted.

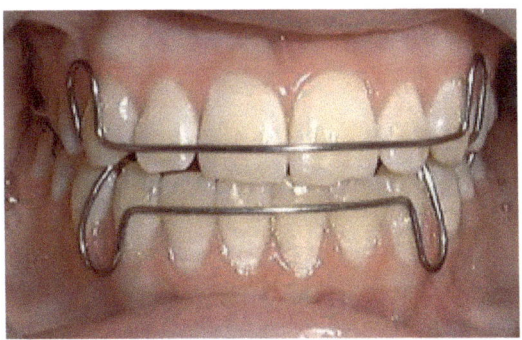

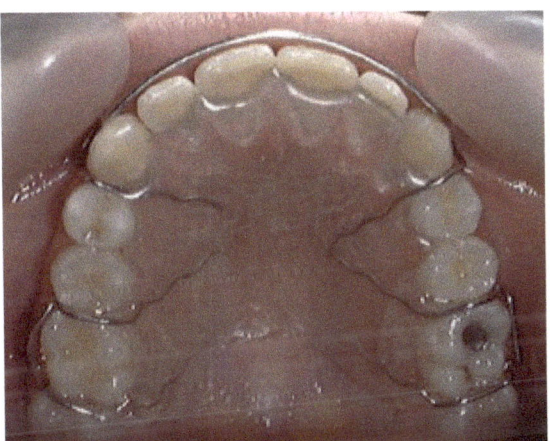

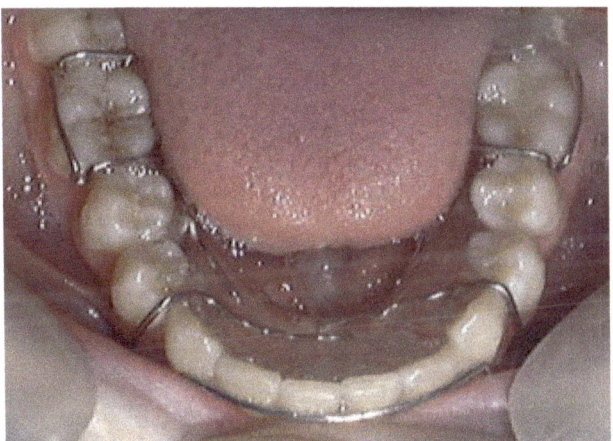

TREATMENT OF DENTAL ASYMMETRY

This 14 year old girl presented a dental asymmetry with upper and lower labial crowding in late mixed dentition. Dental development was later than average as second deciduous molars were still retained. with /3 crowded out of the arch buccally and still to erupt. A panoramic radiograph confirmed the presence of /8 and third molars were absent in the remaining three quadrants. The lower second premolars are unerupted, potentially impacted against the lower first molars with a a pronounced distal angulation. The second deciduous molars showed no sign of shedding and these teeth were extracted, followed by sagittal appliances to maintain space for the second premolars to erupt and create space for the unerupted canine.

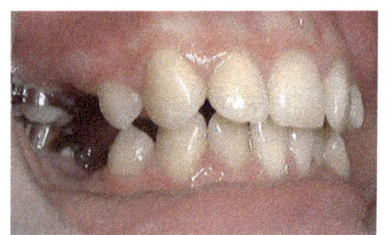 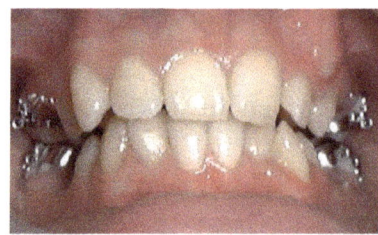 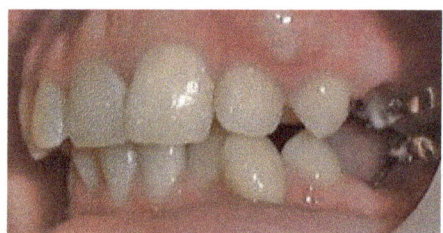

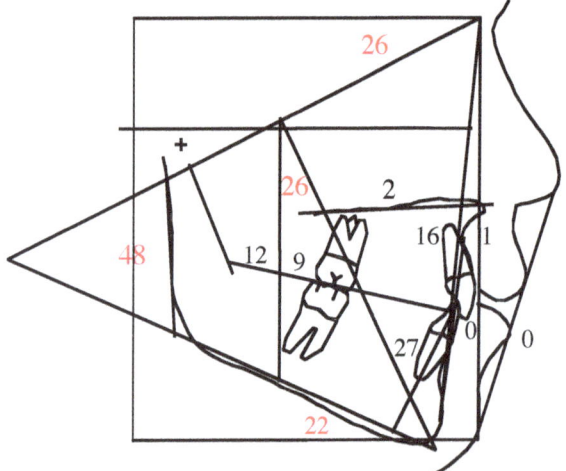 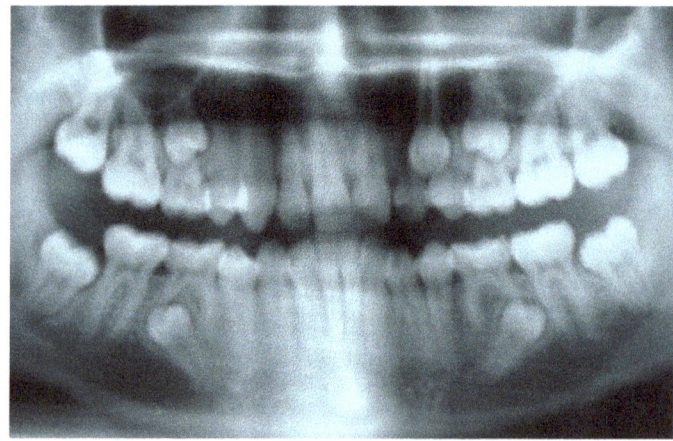

76

A TransForce Sagittal appliance was fitted first to open space to accommodate the blocked out upper canine. This appliance is very effective in correcting dental asymmetries by equalizing the the spaces in the buccal segments to accommodate blocked out premolars or canines. It can be used as the first step in treatment and can then be combined with a fixed appliance. The unerupted premolars were exposed and levered with an elevator by the patient's dentist after removing bone to encourage eruption. The lower arch was developed with a lower Transforce Sagittal appliance in combination with a lower fixed appliance to control the lower incisors.

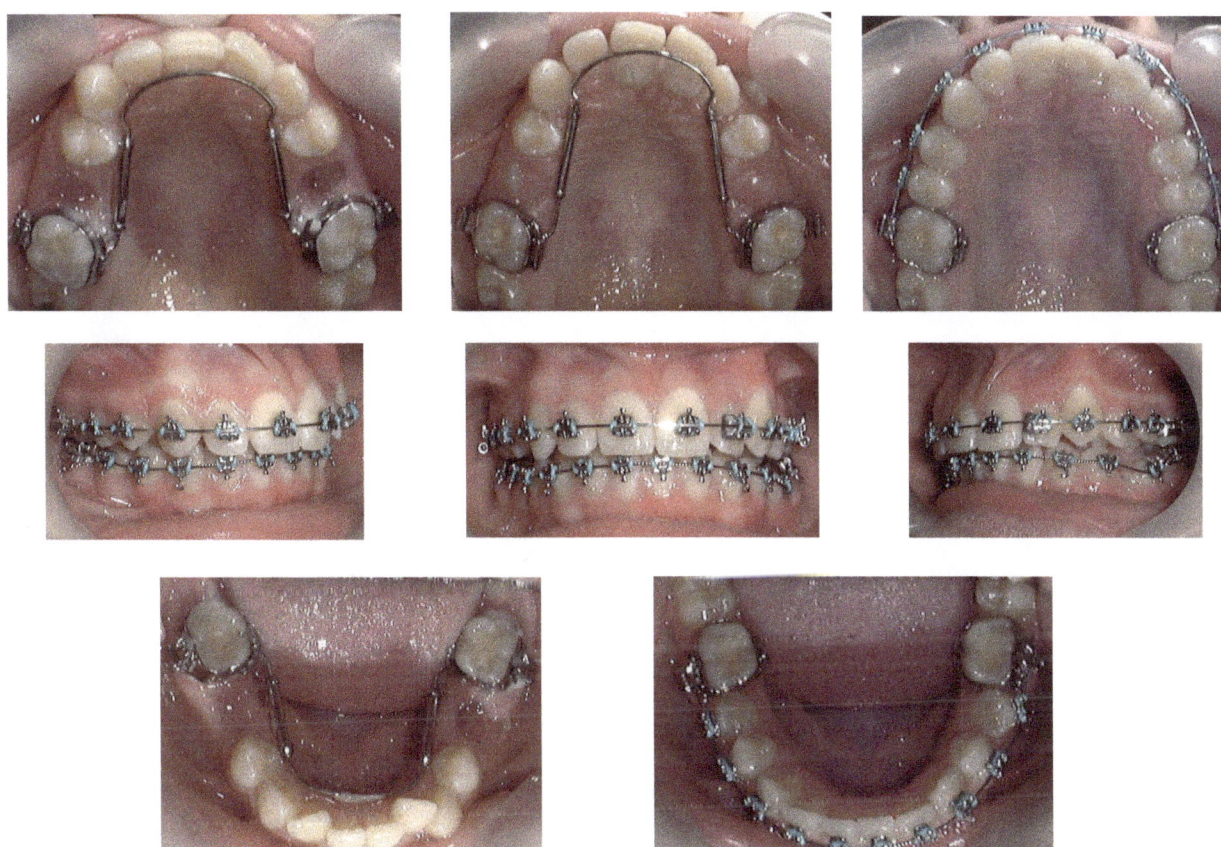

Treatment extended over three years, allowing time for eruption of lower premolars before completing treatment with bonded fixed appliances, followed by removable retainers. Management of the asymmetry was simplified by the ability to equalize spaces in the buccal segments with the sagittal appliance to accommodate the displaced canine.

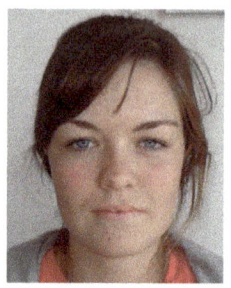 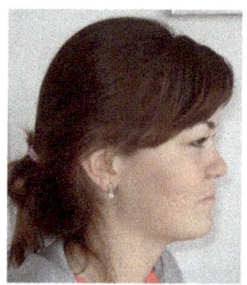 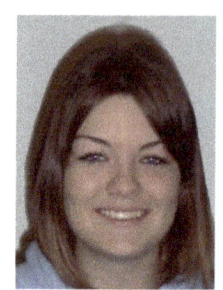

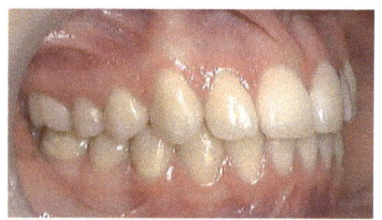 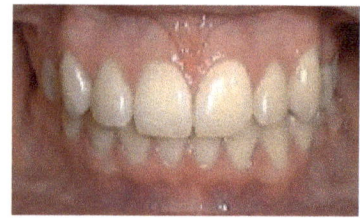 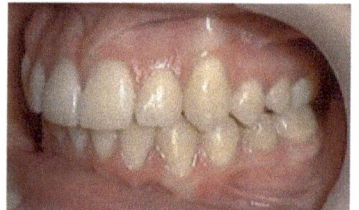

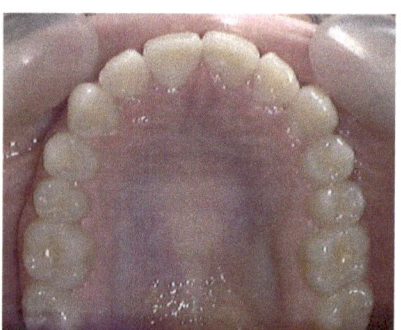 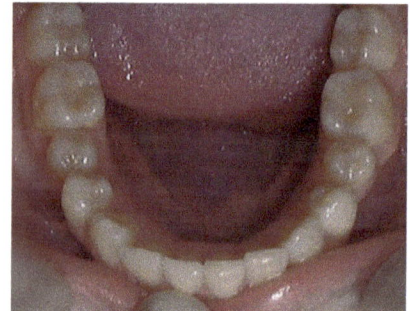

TransForce Orthodontics - Invisible Comfortable & Efficient

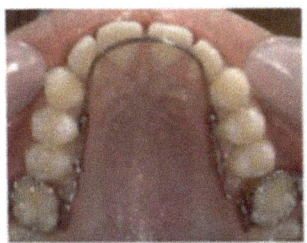 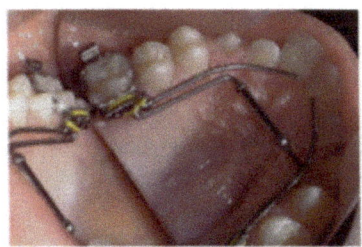

TransForce appliances do not interfere with natural function. The tongue adapts into the palate during treatment as the arches expand. There is an additional advantage that the appliances may remain in place as passive retainers when transverse or sagittal expansion is complete. Pre-activated TransForce appliances require little or no adjustment. The force generated by the Transverse Palatal Expander is 200 grams and expansion is slow and continuous. This minimises the possibility of damage to the periodontal attachment.

4 Months Treatment

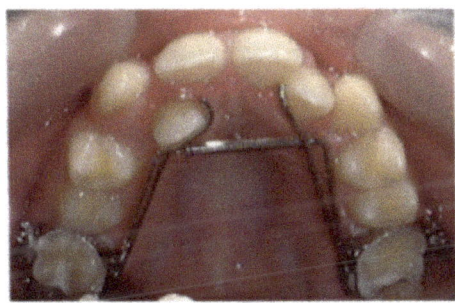 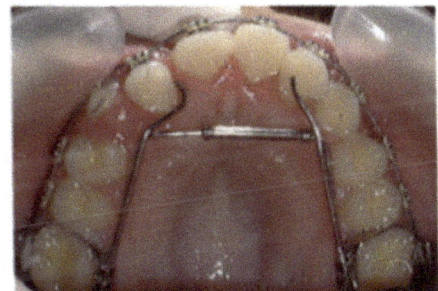

TransForce Orthodontics

TransForce Palatal Expander achieves the objective of delivering physiologic forces within the tolerance of the periodontal tissues by applying a light continuous force of 200 grams for maxillary expansion. This approach resolves anterior crowding in mixed or permanent dentition and has the advantage of expanding the lower arch by bony remodeling of the dento alveolar processes. There is equal expansion of the anterior and posterior segments across the inter-canine and inter-molar width.

The compression unit on the TransForce Transverse appliance is positioned lingual to the incisors across the canine region. This is extremely effective in interceptive treatment to resolve upper and lower labial crowding by increasing the intercanine width before the permanent canines erupt. Alternative appliances for palatal expansion are not as effective in correcting anterior crowding. The anterior wires may be used for additional buccal expansion or labial movement of the incisors if required. The arches may be over - expanded in mixed dentition to encourage the premolars and canines to erupt in a wider arch.

In addition to these biological benefits slow expansion techniques offer a number of clinical advantages. An ideal slow expansion appliance requires minimal adjustment throughout its use, but permits easy adjustment when necessary. It delivers a constant physiologic force until the required expansion is obtained. The appliance is light and comfortable enough to be kept in place for sufficient retention of expansion. Prefabrication eliminates extra appointments and the appliance may be selcted and fitted in the laboratory and delivered ready to fit.

TransForce integrates well with fixed appliances in mixed or permanent dentition. Patients should be informed when two phase treatment is planned and it is recommended that brackets are fitted before the anterior teeth are fully aligned from the lingual aspect.

Guidelines For Case Selection

Indications for TransForce Sagittal Appliance

- Straight profile with retroclined upper and lower incisors and deep overbite

- Upper canines may be crowded buccally and sagittal development may be indicated to resolve labial segment crowding

- Careful case selection is important in the lower arch before selecting a sagittal appliance to advance lower incisors.

- Lower incisors are retroclined and positioned lingually with deep overbite

- Concave Profile: Bimaxillary retrusion with retrusive lips and deep overbite

- Brachyfacial growth pattern with a low mandibular plane angle

- Class II division 2 malocclusion with retroclined incisors and deep overbite

- Class III malocclusion in mixed dentition with retroclined upper incisors and a positive overbite

- TransForce may be integrated with fixed appliances. This is recommended in the lower arch for improved control of lower incisors

- In treatment of crowded arches complete treatment with fixed appliances

- Retention is essential after arch development

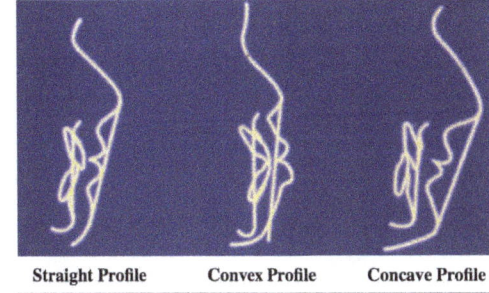

Straight Profile   Convex Profile   Concave Profile

Contra-indications for TransForce Sagittal Appliance

- Bimaxillary protrusion with convex profile, proclined incisors and full lips

- Dolichofacial profile with increased lower facial height

- High mandibular plane angle is unfavourable for sagittal arch development

- Reduced overbite or anterior open bite will worsen if incisors are moved labially

- Severe crowding may require extractions

- For transverse arch development choose the Transverse TransForce

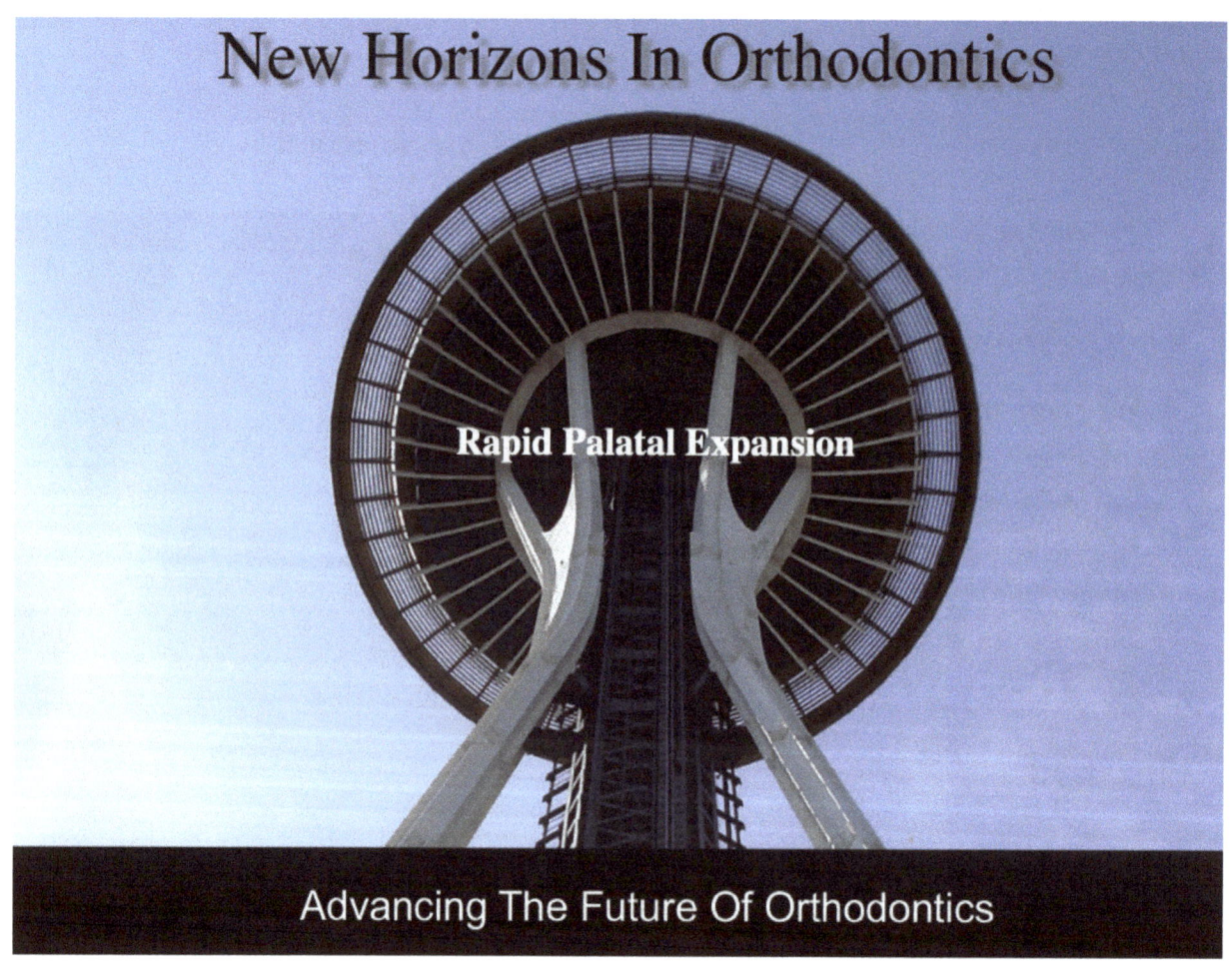

New Horizons In Orthodontics

Rapid Palatal Expansion

Advancing The Future Of Orthodontics

TransForce Orthodontics

Advancing The Future Of Orthodontics

It is time to review the effectiveness of the RPE compared to alternative appliances. Light physiological forces achieve slow expansion at a rate that encourages a cellular response to keep pace with the rate of expansion in the midline suture and alveolar processes. This protocol may prove to be more effective throughout the age range from mixed dentition through adolescence to adult therapy. The fundamental principles of orthopaedic and orthodontic therapy encourage sutural growth in early treatment and move teeth efficiently through alveolar bone, giving time for the natural repair mechanism to encourage growth and development.

In addition to these biological benefits slow expansion techniques offer a number of clinical advantages. An ideal slow expansion appliance requires minimal adjustment throughout its use, but permits easy adjustment when necessary. It delivers a constant physiologic force until the required expansion is obtained. The appliance is light and comfortable enough to be kept in place for sufficient retention of the expansion. Prefabrication eliminates the need for extra appointments. The appliance may be selected and prepared in the laboratory prior to fitting and is delivered ready to fit, but no additional fabrication is required.

As in any expansion procedure, over-expansion is necessary to compensate for the tendency of the posterior teeth to return to their pre-treatment axial inclinations. Once the transverse discrepancy has been corrected, the expander should be kept in place long enough to correct any buccal tipping that occurred earlier in the expansion process.

This description underlines the advantages of TransForce Orthodontics, using preformed, pre-activated appliances to deliver light physiological forces to correct arch form in transverse and sagittal dimensions, followed by retention with the same appliances. TransForce Orthodontics represents a revolution in interceptive treatment using invisible appliances that fit comfortably in the palate to achieve rapid correction in all classes of malocclusion from mixed dentition, through adolescence to adult therapy.

Alternative Techniques For Palatal Expansion

How does the TransForce Palatal Expander compare with alternative techniques for palatal expansion? The Bonded Hyrax Expander is a typical example of the Rapid Palatal Expander. The appliance distrurbs the occlusion and does not permit the tongue to rest in the palate. It occupies the palate and applies heavy forces to split the suture, creating a central diastema.

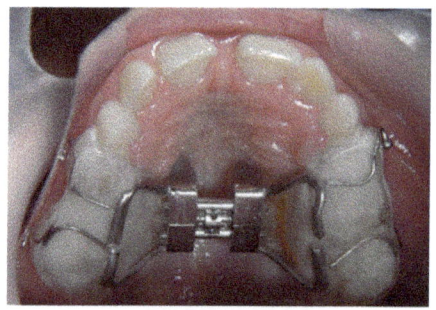

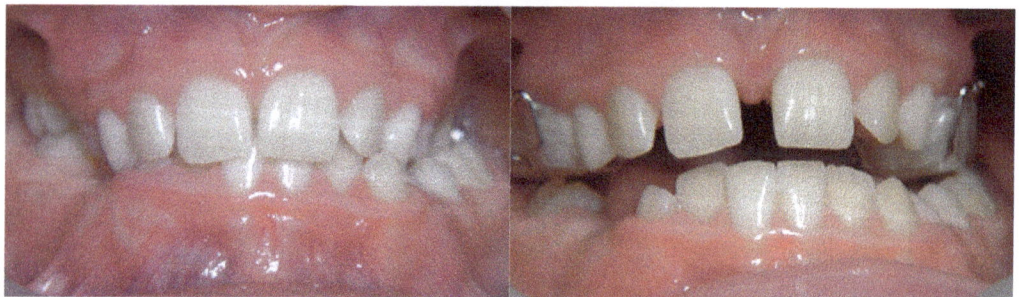

HISTOLOGICAL FINDINGS IN RAPID PALATAL EXPANSION

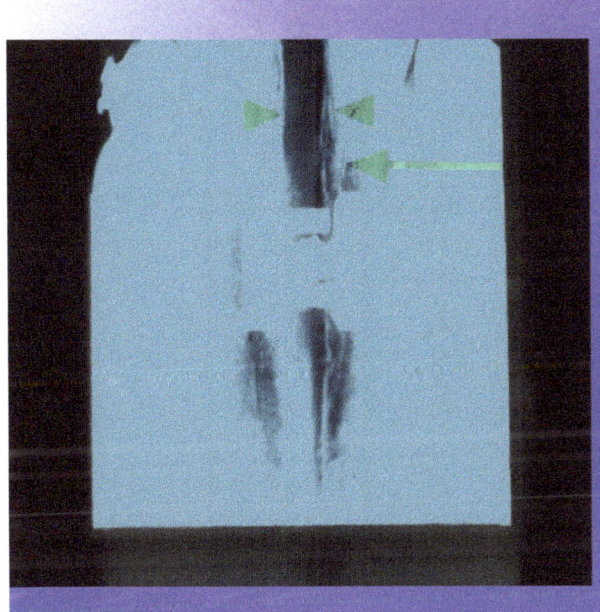

- Free floating bone fragments
- Surrounding micro bone fractures
- Cystic formation
- Vascular disorganization
- Floating fibroblasts
- Spongy bone

This study identified the disadvantages of applying excessive forces to split the midline suture.

- Traumatic forces of 3 to 10 lb + (1.5 to 4.5 KG)
- Pain and discomfort
- Bone fragments and bleeding into the wound
- Repair by spongy bone and fibrous tissue causes relapse
- Buccal dehiscence of bone in adults
- Gingival recession and periodontal damage
- Must be surgically assisted in adults
- Requires laboratory construction

Without surgery when the suture splits heavy forces are applied to the outer alveolar plate. This would result in dehiscence of alveolar bone and loss of the periodontal attachment. Three stages are necessary in a protocol for Rapid Palatal expansion in adult therapy

- Pre-surgical orthodontics
- Maxillary alveolar surgery
- Post surgical orthodontics
- Lengthy and expensive treatment

Is there an optimal force for sutural expansion?
Liu, Opperman, Kyung, Buschang   A.J.O.D.O. 2011, 139 pp 446 - 455

This title refers to an animal study with young rabbits reported in the AJODO in 2011. Animal studies have contributed significantly to our knowledge of orthodontics and dentofacial orthopaedics. The purpose of this study was to establish the causal relationships between expansion force magnitudes, sutural separation, and sutural bone formation.

Within the limits of this study, sutural bone formation is directly related to the amount of sutural separation, which is in turn related to the amount of force applied. The results suggest that there is a level of induced sutural separation that provides the greatest amount of bone formation. The conclusions were as follows:

- Higher force levels produce greater sepration but do not produce more bone
- They have greater relapse potential after forces are removed
- Require longer periods of retention
- Without retention, relapse can amount to 45% of sutural separtion

Computer-aided design and manufacture of hyrax devices: Can we really go digital?

Graf, Cornelis, Gameiro, & Cattaneo. AJODO, 152, 870-874, 2017

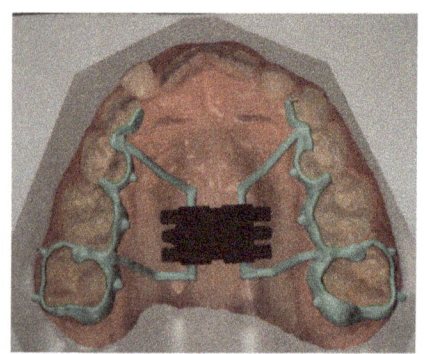
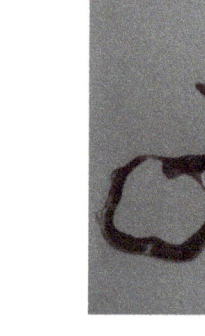

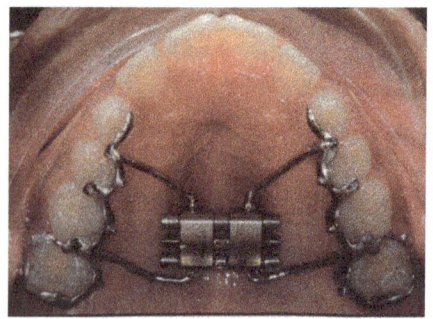
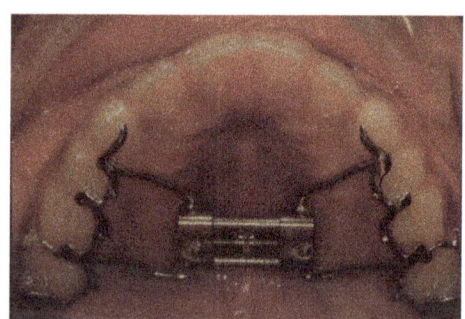

Computer-aided design and manufacture of hyrax devices: Can we really go digital?
Graf, Cornelis, Gameiro, & Cattaneo. AJODO, 152, 870-874, 2017

It is claimed that this technique advances the Rapid Palatal Expander into the digital age. However it is doubtful if this represents progress in terms of technology. Accidents have been reported in the literature and this problem has not been resolved.

Ingestion of a RPE activation key: why do these accidents still happen?
Pantuzo, Nunes, Pires. European Paediatric Dentistry, Feb,2017
Accidental ingestion of a rapid maxillary expander activation key in a cardiac patient.

Activation of the RPE expects a non professional to place a pin in the mouth to activate the appliance every day, taking no account of the dexterity or eyesight of the person allocated to perform this task. Palatal damage or ingestion of the key continue to happen.

Orthodontic laboratories have observed difficulties when the scew is turned backwards in trying to remove it from the mouth resulting in no progress or breakage of the screw. In spite of using digital technology to customise these appliances, the appliance mechanism is not satisfactory, taking into account the danger of acccidents and periodontal damage from heavy traumatic forces. In addition this computer generated technique is expensive compared to pre-activated TransForce appliances delivering light physiological forces.

The RPE is a dinosaur in the method of activation as a professional mechanism.

Nitinol Palatal Expander

The Nitinol Palatal Expander is an alternative to the Rapid Palatal Expander, but must be selected and adjusted carefully to avoid tooth movement that tip the teeth excessively. Failure to select the correct size of this appliance can cause periodontal damage. The upper molars and premolars are overexpanded in this case. This would cause gingival recession in an adult.

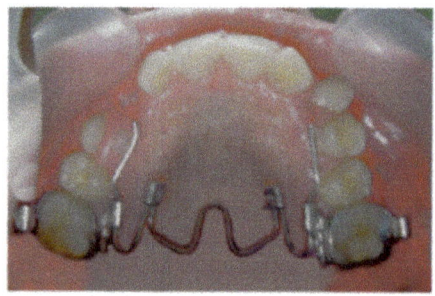 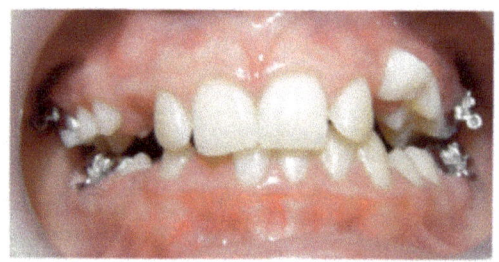

Occlusal X-rays will seldom show palatal separation during slow expansion procedures. The gradual rate of expansion maintains tissue integrity and elicits a physiologic response that allows a deposition along the suture to keep pace. Consequently an unsightly midline gap can be avoided and the arch length gained can be used to align ectopic canines and premolars.

As in any expansion procedure, over expansion is necessary to compensate for the tendency of posterior teeth to upright. The expander should remain in place to retain as the occlusion settles.

Slow Maxillary Expansion with Nickel Titanium
Roberto Murzban DDS, Ravindra Nanda BDS, MDS, PHD

In animal studies slow expansion procedures have demonstrated orthopaedic effects similar to RPE. Histological examination suggests that sutural separation does occur, but at a rate that maintains the integrity of the maxilllary sutures by allowing for bone remodeling. Clinical studies of human patients in the deciduous or early mixed dentition substantiate these findings. Maxillary width increases ranged from 3.8 mm to 8.7 mm with slow expansion of as much as 1 mm per week using 900 grams of force with the Ni-Ti maxillary expander.

Storey recommends slow expansion at 0.5 to 1 mm per week to allow for "physiological sutural adjustments", which elicit less trauma and a greater repair response compared to rapid maxillary expansion. Ekstrom reports that slowly expanded sutures become well organised in 30 days and are well established with mineralized tissue by three months.

Slow expansion has been found to promote greater post-expansion stability, given an adequate retention period. Furthermore, in comparison of slow expansion with a quad helix and RPE Zachrisson concluded that periodontal breakdown on the buccal aspects of posterior teeth occurred infrequently in both groups, but the few patients who exhibited some attachment loss were in the RPE group.

The Nickel Titanium Expander provides a viable alternative to rapid expansion for correction of transverse discrepancie. Incorporation into an existing fixed appliance eliminates a separate laboratory phase and extra appointments for impressions, adjustments and rebanding molars afer removal. The buccal molar attachments are available for use with intrusion arches, utility arches or comprehensive fixed appliances.

TransForce Palatal Expander

Compared to these techniques the TransForce palatal expander is simple and unobtrusive. TransForce appliances are invisible and comfortable to wear and apply physiological forces without pain or damage to the supporting bone. Low forces of 200 grams are applied to the buccal segments so that the force applied to individual teeth is reduced to approximately 50 grams.

These are the force levels recommended by Ricketts in the Bioprogressive Philosophy. This was subsequently verified by periodontologists as the optimum force levels for tooth movement in palatal expansion to avoid unwanted side effects of buccal dehiscence of alveolar bone in the outer alveolar plate. Periodontologists review the long term effects of orthodontic treatment. We must take into account their observations relating to gingival recession and periodontal support out of retention. Early intervention is ideal in treatment of maxillary contraction. It encourages the permanent successors to erupt in a wider arch form.

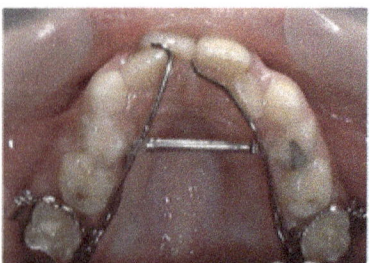 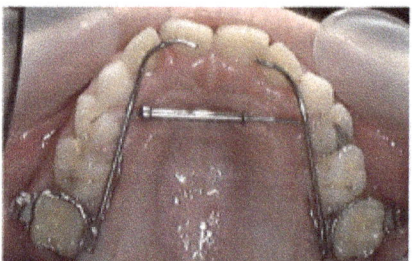 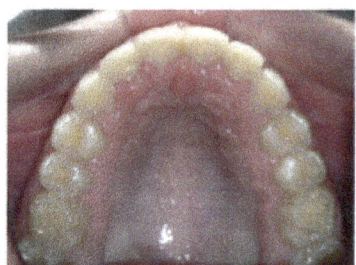

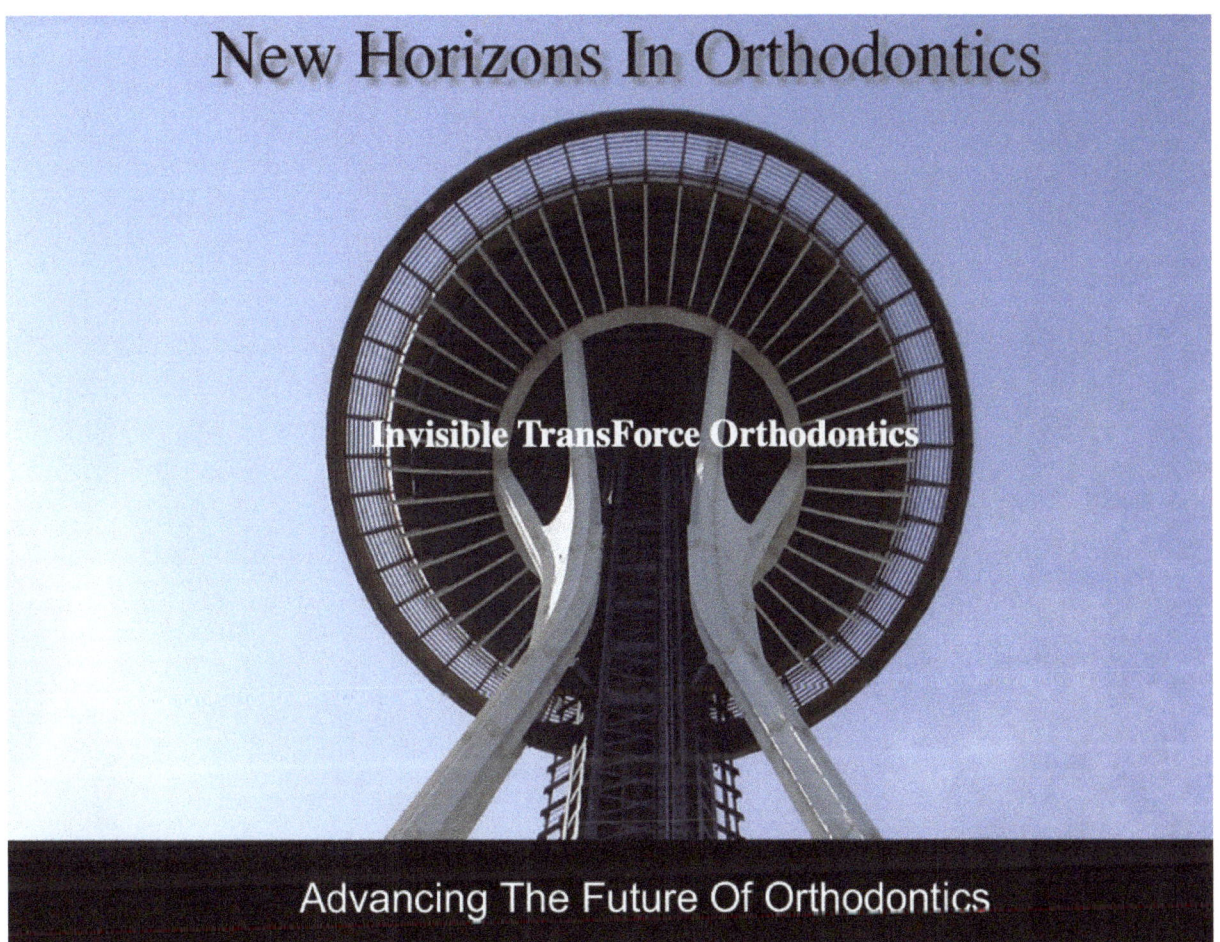

New Horizons In Orthodontics

Invisible TransForce Orthodontics

Advancing The Future Of Orthodontics

TransForce Orthodontics - Invisible Comfortable & Efficient

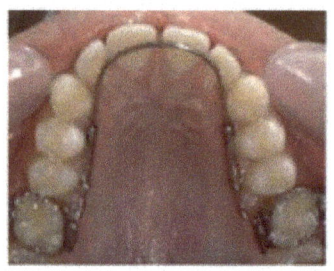 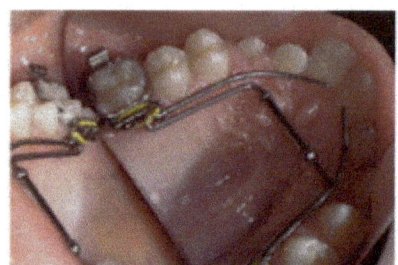

TransForce appliances do not interfere with natural function. The tongue adapts into the palate during treatment as the arches expand. There is an additional advantage that the appliances may remain in place as passive retainers when transverse or sagittal expansion is complete. Pre-activated TransForce appliances require little or no adjustment. The force generated by the Transverse Palatal Expander is 200 grams and expansion is slow and continuous. This minimises the possibility of damage to the periodontal attachment.

4 Months Treatment

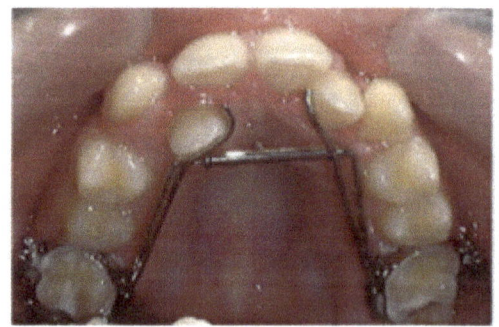 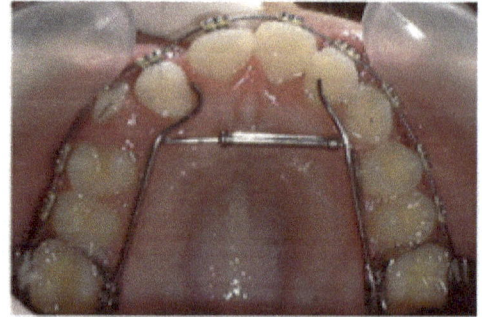

Invisible Orthodontic Appliances

An important aspect of contemporary orthodontic technique is to ensure that control of treatment planning and delivery of the highest standards of orthodontic treatment remains in the hands of trained specialists. There is a danger with the advance of computer technology that diagnosis and treatment planning may be presented directly to the public by untrained technicians working on computers with no direct contact with the patient.

It is already evident that a direct appeal to the public to subscribe to invisible appliances is largely based on the evaluation of a scanned model of the dentition. The prospect of self diagnosis is a small step away from an unprofessional approach with the problems that may present for unsuspecting patients.

It is important to preserve the principles of Ricketts Bioprogressive Philosophy. Treatment planning is based on facial growth and development. Utility arches enable interceptive treatment in mixed dentition when appropriate to resolve severe malocclusions before the permanent teeth erupt.

Interceptive techniques using invisibe appliances are increasingly important for the orthodontist in order to compete with the growing trend for invisible appliances. The days of brackets and braces may be numbered and we must develop alternative techniques that appeal to the public.

TransForce Orthodontics is a technique for the professional based on invisible appliances in the hands of the orthodontist. This competes favourably with computer generated systems designed to correct malocclusion in the permaent dentition. Interceptive treatment is increasingly important from mixed dentition to adult therapy. TransForce Orthodontics offers an alternative approach with excellent potential in adult therapy using invisible appliances prescribed by the orthodontist.

TransForce Orthodontics

TransForce Palatal Expander acheives the objective of delivering physiologic forces within the tolerance of the periodontal tissues by applying a light continuous force of 200 grams for maxillary expansion. This approach resolves anterior crowding in mixed or permanent dentition and has the advantage of expanding the lower arch by bony remodeling of the dento alveolar processes. There is equal expansion of the anterior and posterior segments across the inter-canine and inter-molar width.

The compression unit on the TransForce Transverse appliance is positioned ligual to the incisors across the canine region. This is extremely effective in interceptive treatment to resolve upper and lower labial crowding by increasing the intercanine width before the permanent canines erupt. Alternative appliances for palatal expansion are not as effective in correcting anterior crowding. The anterior wires may be used for additional buccal expansion or labial movement of the incisors if required. The arches may be over - expanded in mixed dentition to encourage the premolars and canines to erupt in a wider arch.

In addition to these biological benefits slow expansion techniques offer a number of clinical advantages. An ideal slow expansion appliance requires minimal adjustment throughout its use, but permits easy adjustment when necessary. It delivers a constant physiologic force until the required expansion is obtained. The appliance is light and comfortable enough to be kept in place for sufficient retention of expansion. Prefabrication eliminates extra appointments and the appliance may be selcted and fitted in the laboratory and delivered ready to fit.

TransForce integrates well with fixed appliances in mixed or permanent dentition. Patients should be informed when two phase treatment is planned and it is recommended that brackets are fitted before the anterior teeth are fully aligned from the lingual aspect.

Maxillary Transverse Expander

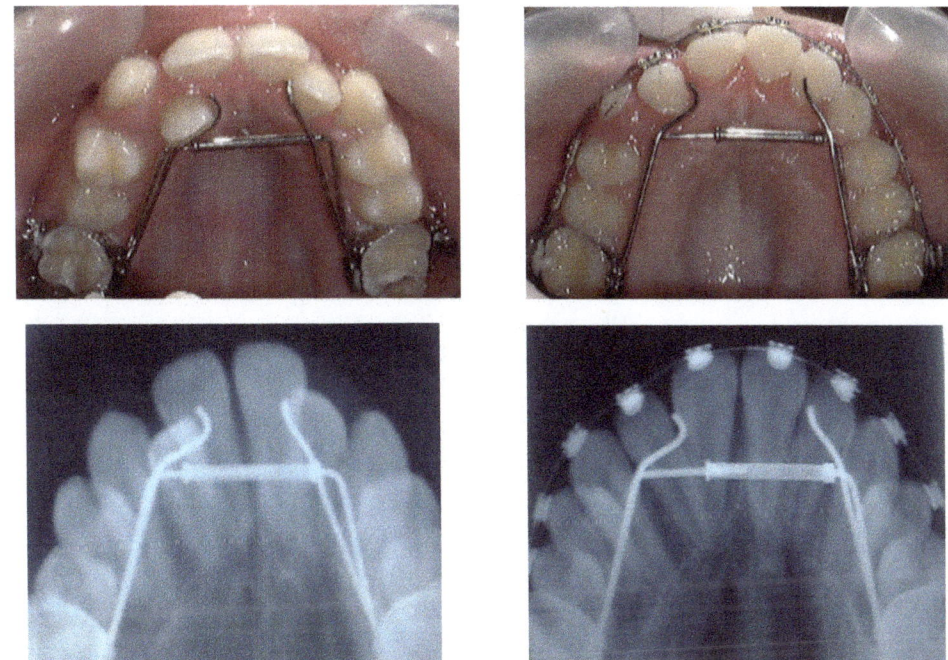

4 months treatment

Mandibular Transverse Expander

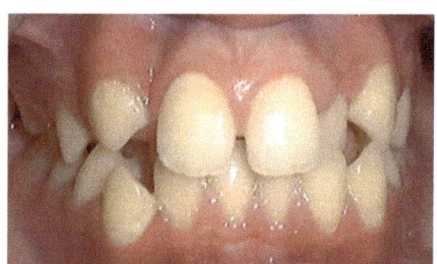

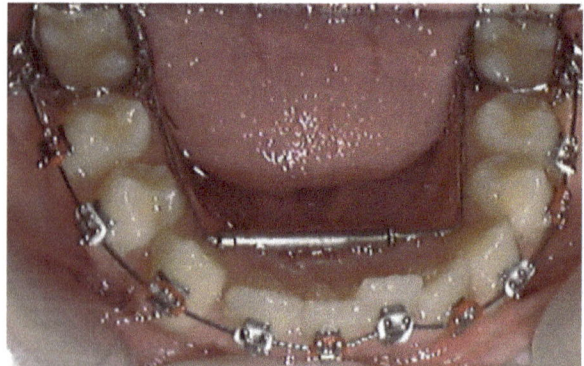 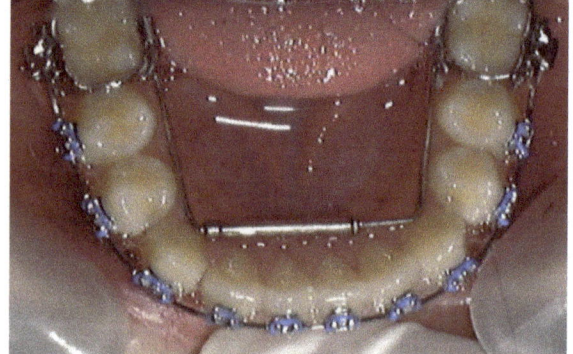

6 months treatment

18 months treatment

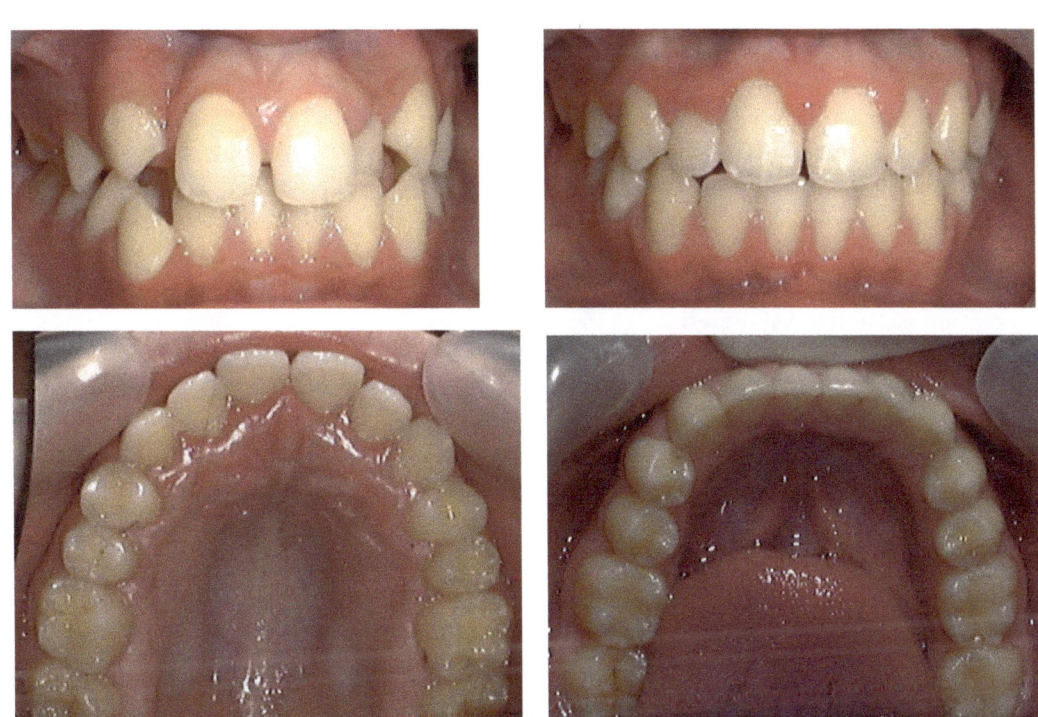

TransForce Sagittal Expander is designed to increase arch length by applying light physiologic forces to advance the anterior teeth. It is indicated when the incisors are retroclined with deep overbite for patients with a flat profile or bimaxillary retrusion. Reciprocal forces are applied to the molars and the anterior teeth and the force levels favour labial movement of the anterior teeth.

Molar width increases as the sagittal appliance expands due to the angulation of the compresion units. Addditional transverse expansion may be acheived by activating the anterior extension wires to move premolars and canines or deciduous teeth buccally if required. This may be indicated in mixed dentition to over expand the arch in order to encourage premolars and canines to erupt in a wider arch.

Correction of Dental Asymmetry

The Transforce Sagittal Expander is extremely effective at correcting dental asymmetry by equalizing the space available for eruption of premolars and canines on each side. When the appliance is inserted it is more compressed on the side that has more crowding and as it expands it corrects the asymmetry and accommodates the erupting teeth on both sides. This is effective in both arches and it is a unique advantage of the pre-activated Transforce Sagittal Expander that does not apply to any other appliance.

In conclusion this report outlines the advantages of pre-activated Transverse and Sagittal TransForce appliances compared to alternative appliance systems for palatal and lingual expansion in both dental arches. TransForce Orthodontics delivers three waay expansion and is effective from mixed dentition through adolescence to adult therapy in all classes of malocclusion.

Sagittal Appliances
6 Months Treatment

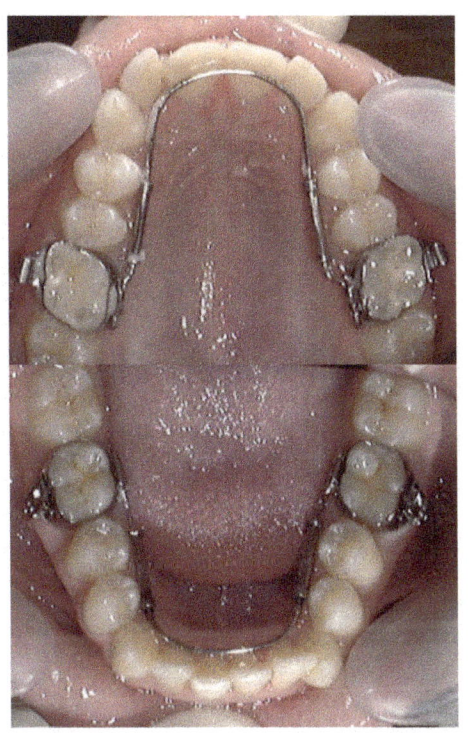
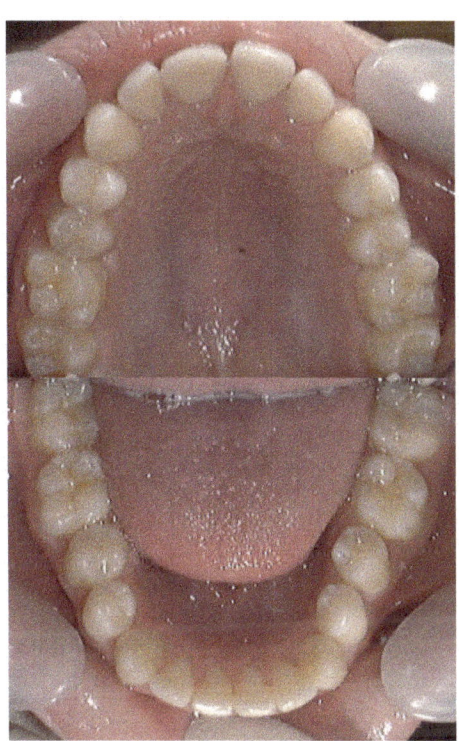

TransForce Orthodontics is equally effective from mixed dentition through to adult therapy

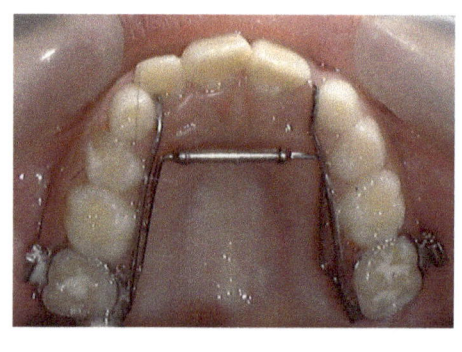
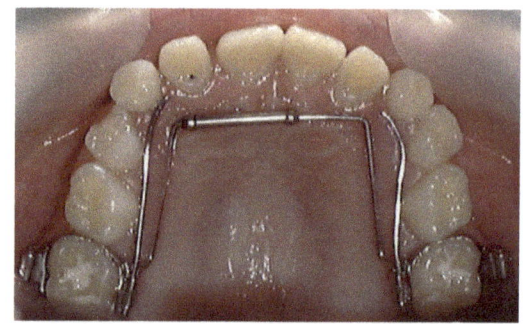
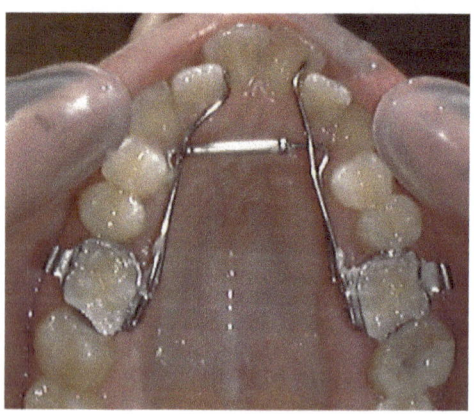
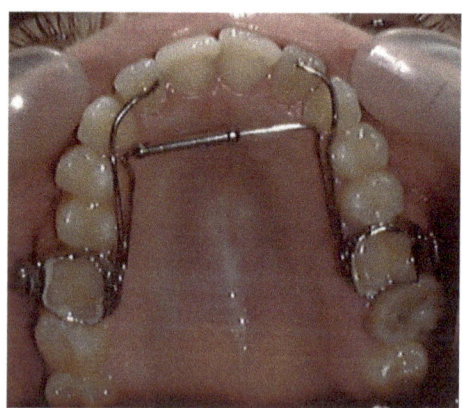

Treatment of a Unilateral Crossbite

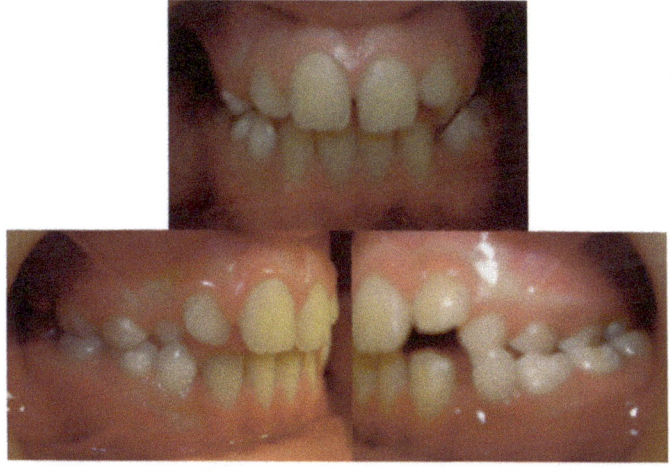

Before Treatment - A Four Tooth Smile!

Next Visit - Crossbite Corrected

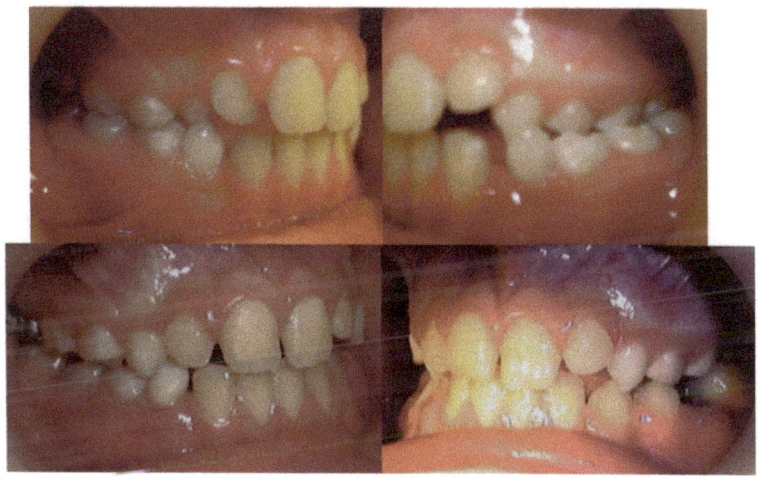

10 weeks Later

Arch Development

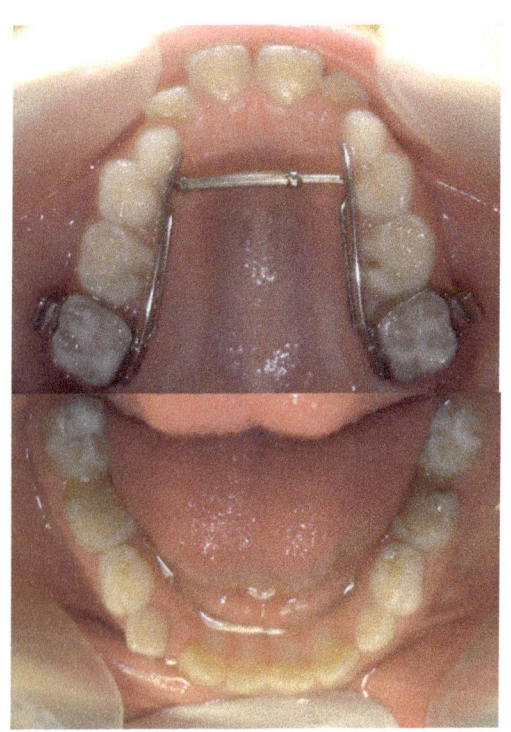
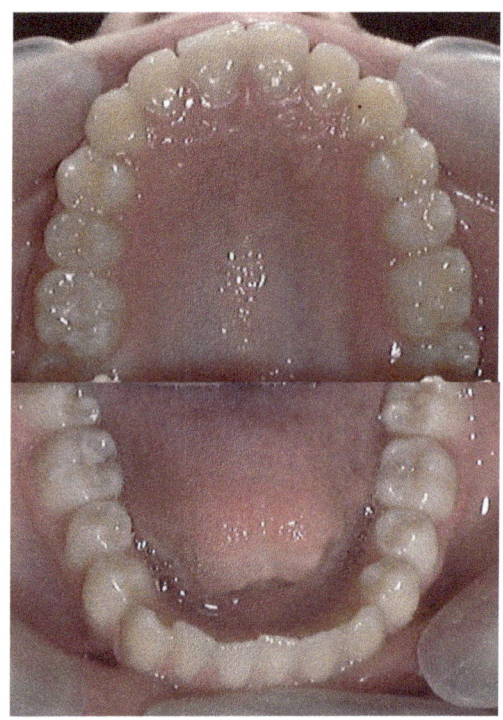

Second Phase

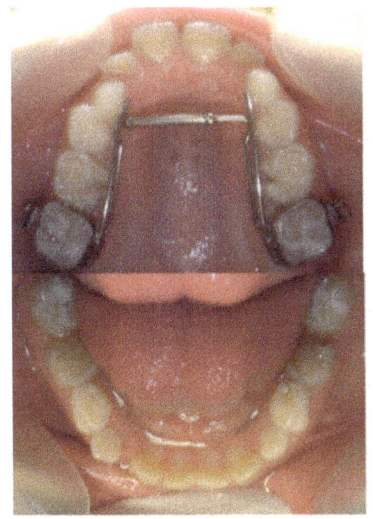

Mixed Dentition

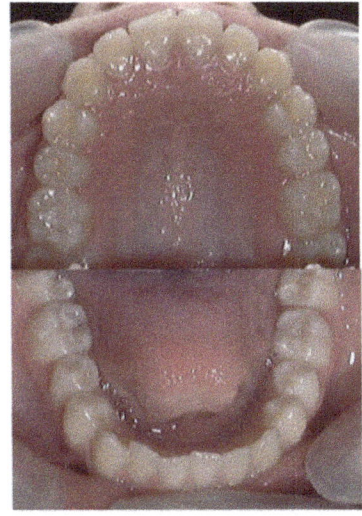

Permanent Dentition

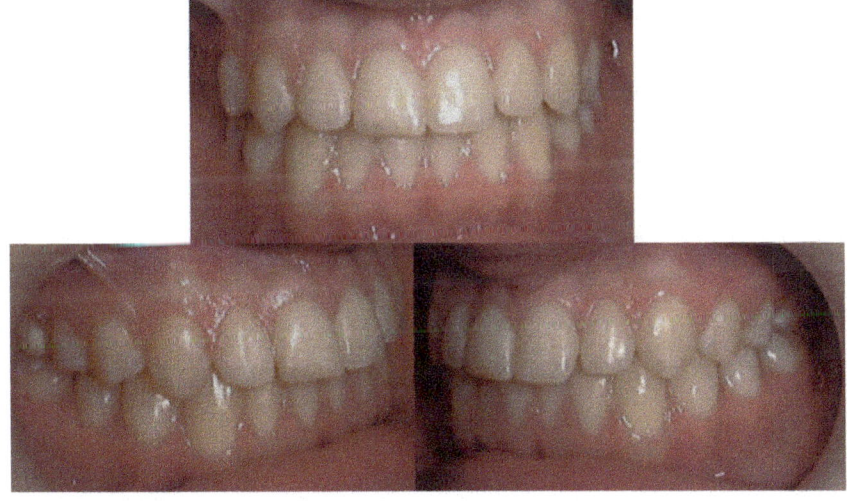

After Treatment

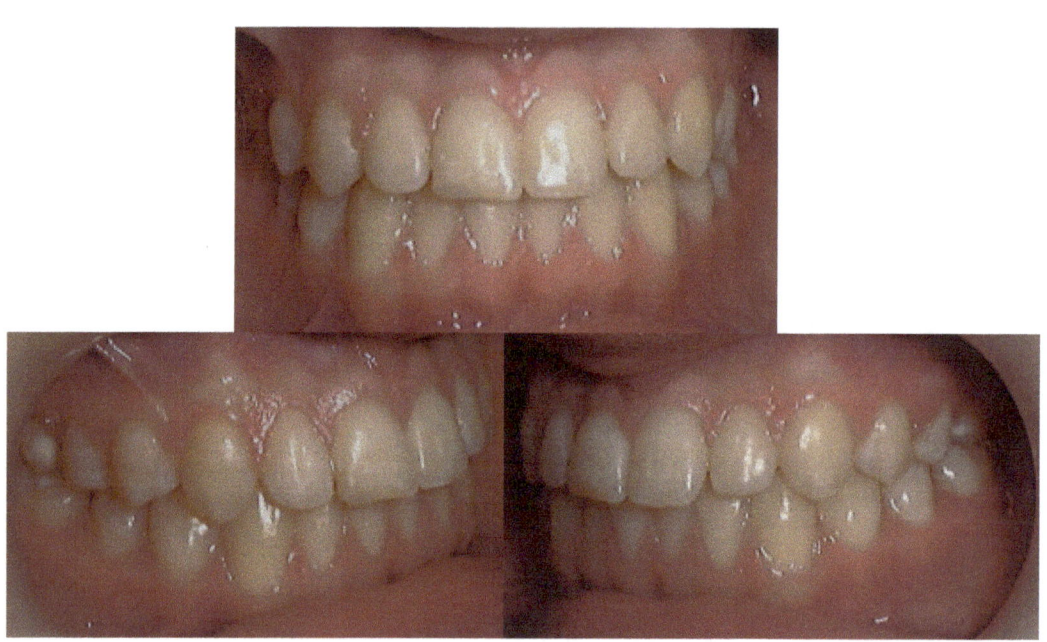

An Eight Tooth Smile!

TransForce Orthodontics is equally effective from mixed dentition through to adult therapy

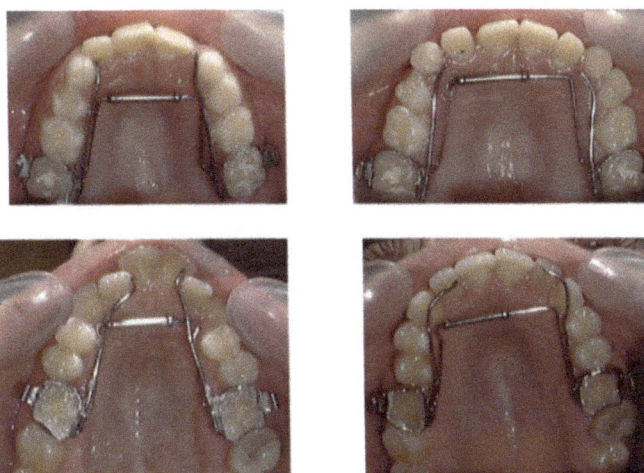

Mixed To Permanent Dentition

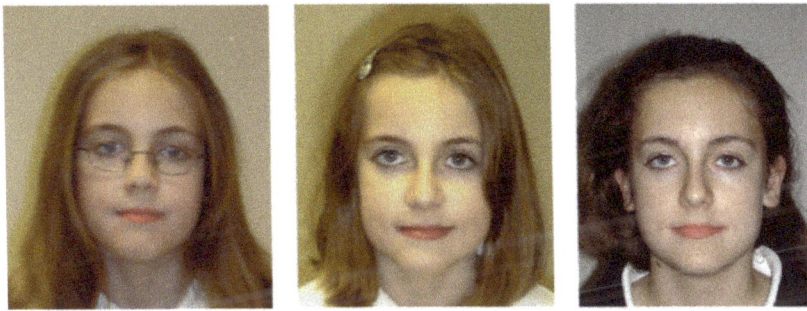

The maxilla is wider after arch development

TransForce Orthodontics

- Non compliance - Fixed/Removable
- Sagittal and Transverse appliances
- Invisible upper & lower appliances
- Low continuous forces reduce discomfort & trauma
- Little or no adjustment required after fitting
- Reduce chair time by 50% !!!
- Integrates with labial & lingual brackets
- Integrates with Invisible Appliances
- Ideal for adult treatment

Try it - You'll like it !

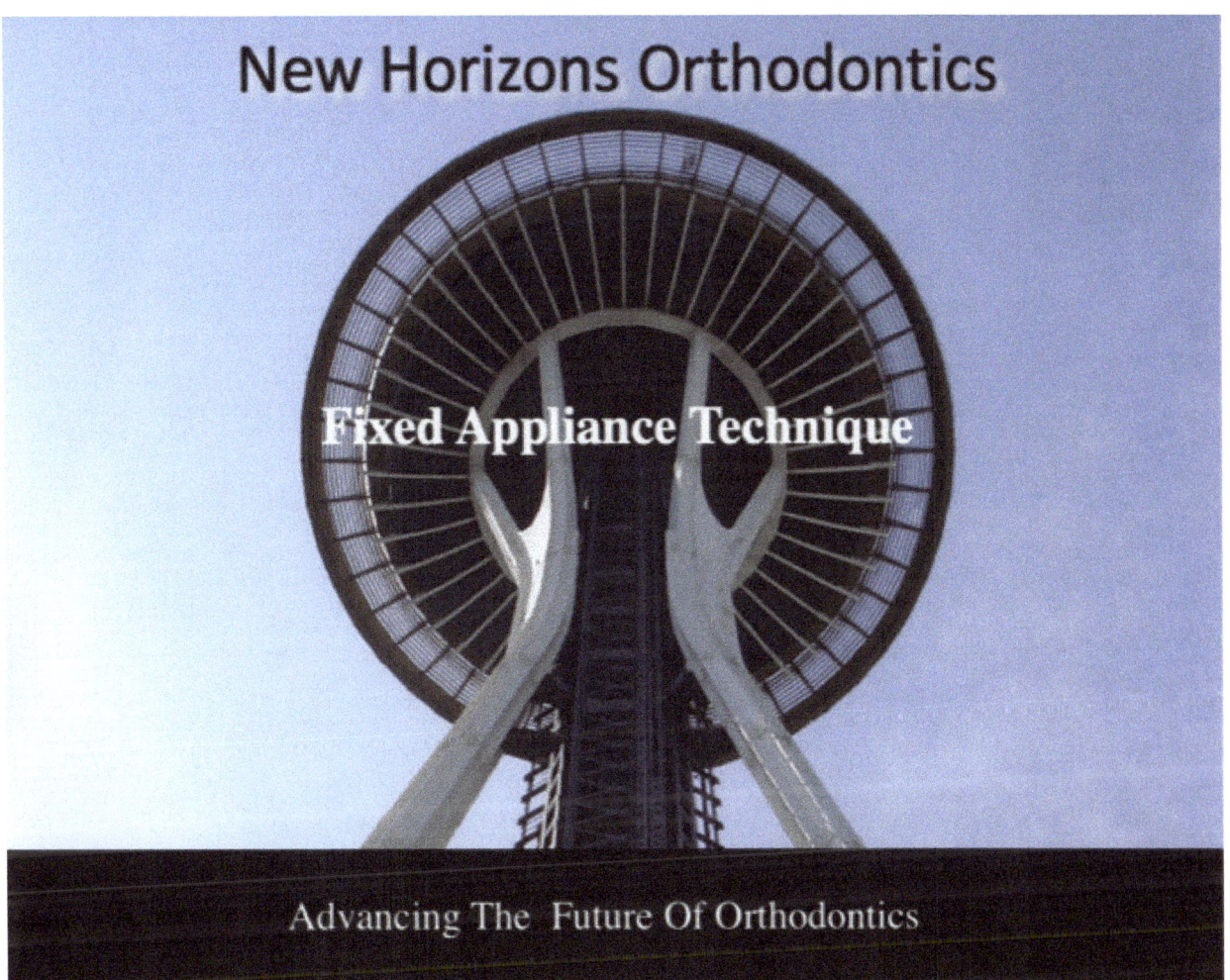

Advances In Fixed Appliance Technique

Current orthodontic techniques have benefitted from technological change in the development of increasingly sophisticated bracket systems. Allegiance to a specific bracket system continues to be a strong characteristic in the selection of brackets used in a specific practice.

Increasingly market pressures determine the bracket system of choice in many orthodontic practices. There is fierce competition among Orthodontic supply companies, which attempt to seduce students to use their system by offering to supply materials free to orthodontic training establishments in order to influence students before they graduate and to capture their allegiance from cradle to grave. Teachers and students should be aware of this, and should not assume that any system is the best without testing the market by using alternatives.

In the days of multi-band techniques it was virtually impossible to change the bracket system in clinical practice, due to the large inventory of pre-welded bands. It was a major inconvenience, not to mention a large investment to consider adopting a new technique.

Direct bonding of brackets has changed that. It is now possible to purchase brackets for an individual patient or in packs of five. There is no need for a young student to confine their experience to a single bracket prescription. Provided the same size slot is used it is perfectly feasible to test the market to determine which bracket system or prescription suits the individual orthodontist, or more appropriately, the individual patient.

It is possible to evaluate bracket systems before purchasing large case loads of brackets. Try the finger test! Pick up a model with brackets and arch wires and run your finger round the arch. How smooth are the brackets? That is what your patient will experience. If you are aware that the brackets are rather prominent, they are high profile, and will be more uncomfortable for patients, especially in the early stages of treatment, but perhaps throughout treatment for sensitive patients. If the brackets are smooth they are low profile, and that may help your reputation. All brackets are not equal!

The main theme of this book, showing the evolution of fixed appliances over the last 50 years is to demonstrate the choice of techniques that is available and to encourage young orthodontists to realize that there is no panacea in orthodontic technique. Rather there is constant evolution. It is the nature of marketing that companies produce new products every year, that are improved versions of what has gone before, but there is a limit to the improvements in bracket systems that basically produce very similar results by orthodontic correction.

A review of the patient records in this book will confirm that the patients selected for fixed appliances have Class I malocclusion or mild Class II or Class III malocclusion. This is because the mechanics of conventional orthodontic techniques are essentially designed to treat Class I malocclusion or patients with only a mild skeletal discrepancy.

The exceptions are some severe dolichofacial patients who would not respond to functional correction and receive camouflage extraction therapy, and younger patients who are offered arch development to improve constricted arches to improve function and guide eruption of permanent teeth into favourable arch form and thus simplify the finishing stages of treatment.

In this section the author shows patients treated with bracket systems he currently uses, with examples of extraction and non extraction therapy. They have suited his protocol and have stood the test of time by producing a consistent standard of results with the minimum of inconvenience. A large range of bracket designs and prescriptions are available at this stage of development of orthodontic techniques.

ELITE® OPTI-MIM® MINI-TWIN BRACKETS
Ortho Organizers

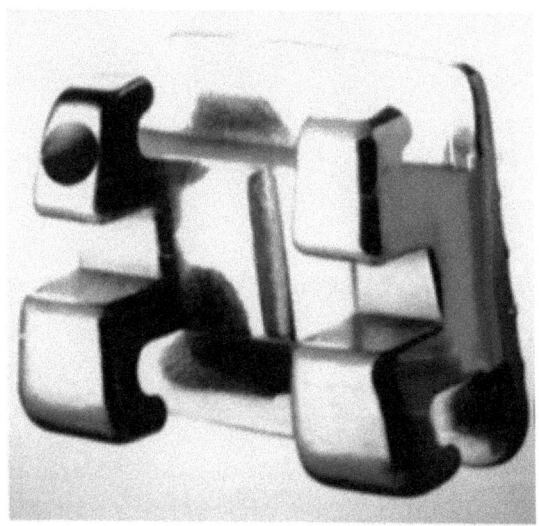

Twin edgewise brackets were originally developed in the Tweed era to fit on first molar bands, and the system was later extended to the remaining teeth to improve rotational control compared to the narrow edgewise bracket. The MIM process (Metal Injection Moulding) for casting brackets revolutionized the manufacture of orthodontic brackets. This process was adopted by all the major orthodontic companies.

This allowed increasingly sophisticated designs to be produced. Opti-Mim Mini-Twin brackets are designed to match the anatomical shape of the tooth with a vertical scribe line along the long axis of the tooth for accurate placement. They have bevelled edges on the slot for easy placement of the archwire and are low profile, with rounded tie-wings to improve patient comfort.

Elite® Opti Mim® is a registered trademark of Ortho Organizers

TREATMENT OF A MILD MALOCCLUSION
Opti-Mim® Mini-Twin Brackets

This 12 year old girl presents a mild Class I malocclusion and is treated with Opti-Mim Mini Twin Brackets, which are an excellent example of a popular bracket system. This sequence of photographs records a typical series of archwire changes as we progress from flexible round wires to level and align the teeth. The initial arch wire is .014" Nickel Titanium.

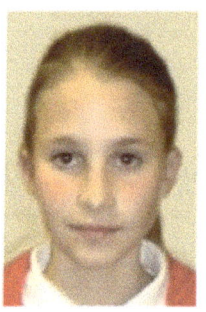
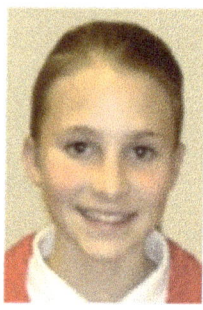
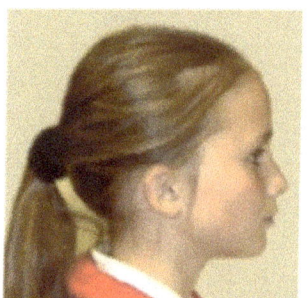

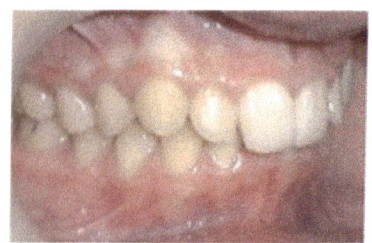
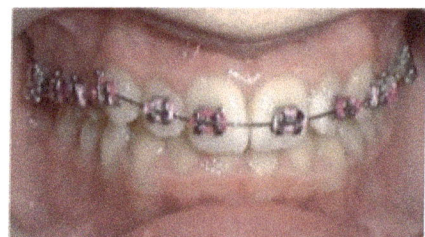
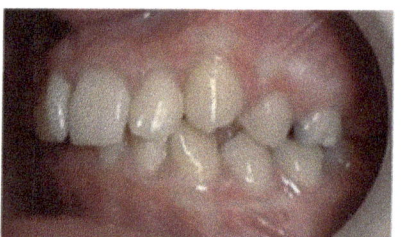

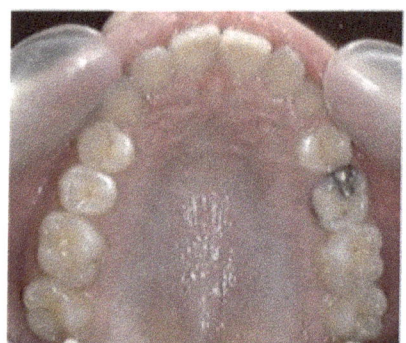
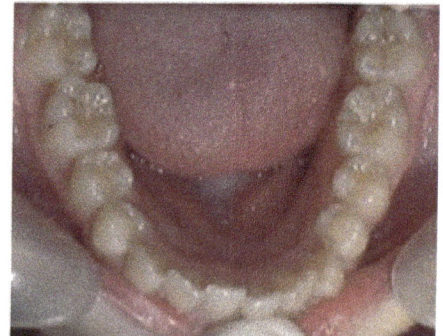

The upper fixed appliance was fitted first and at the next visit it was an advantage to fit a TransForce appliance for transverse expansion in the lower arch to unlock the malocclusion. The Transforce appliance was worn for   3 months to create space to resolve lower labial crowding.

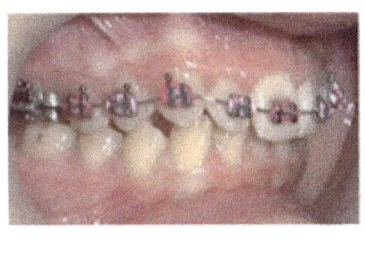 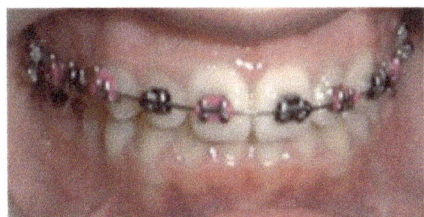 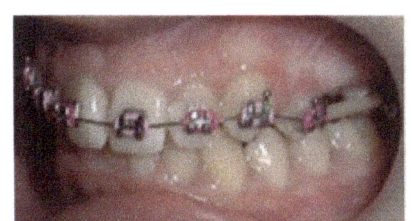

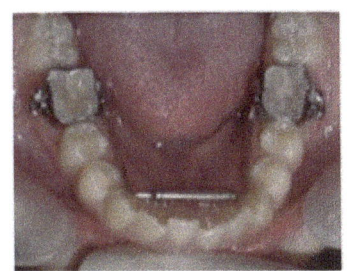 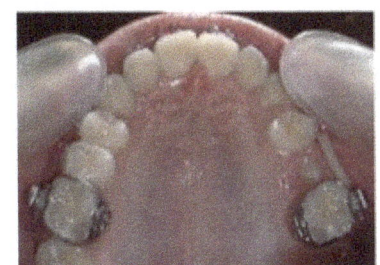 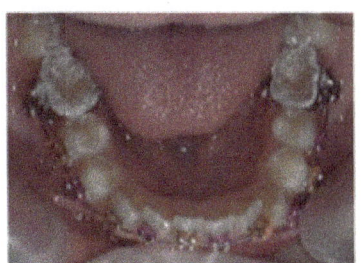

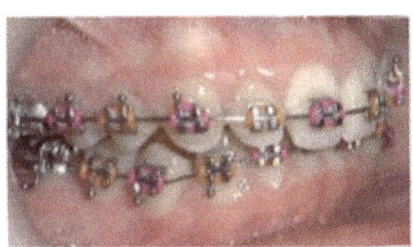 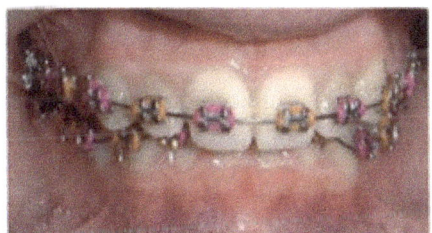 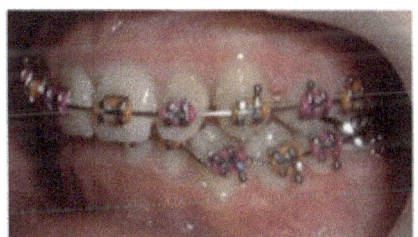

This young lady is very fashion conscious and she rings the changes in colour combinations throughout her treatment, This is fun and she enjoys spending a great deal of time deciding which colours to have this month! After 8 months' treatment the upper arch is levelled and aligned and having worked through from .014 Ni-Ti to .016X.016 and .016 X .022 Ni-Ti wires, an .017 X .025 S.S. upper oval arch is fitted. The lower arch has been aligned with supercable and advances to .016 Ni- Ti.

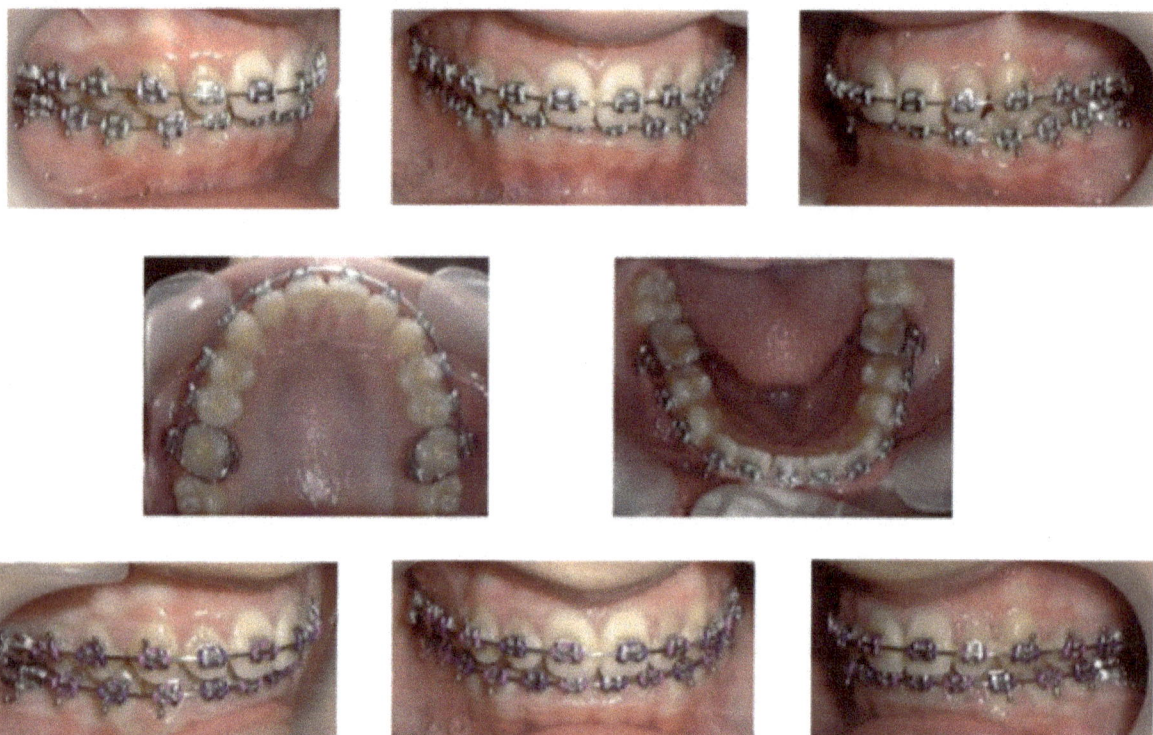

The next step is to progess to an .019 X .025 SS oval upper arch, and the lower arch progresses through .016X .022 Ni Ti to .017 X .025 NiTi after one year to level the lower arch. At the next visit a lower .019 X .025 SS. oval arch is fitted as a finishing arch.

Treatment has extended over a period of 22 months. It does not necessarily take less time to correct a mild malocclusion. The 2/ is not an ideal shape and the patient's dentist, Dr Carvalho, is consulted before we decide on a composite build up to re-shape this tooth.

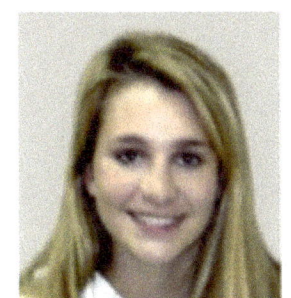 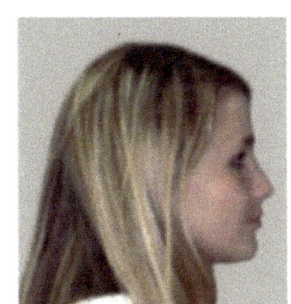

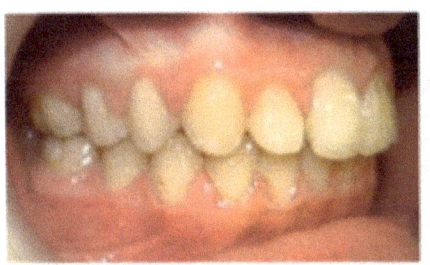 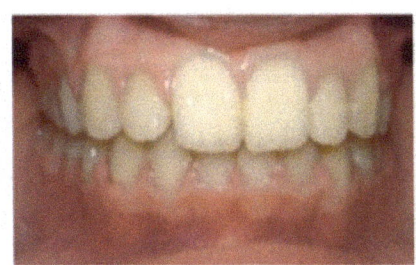 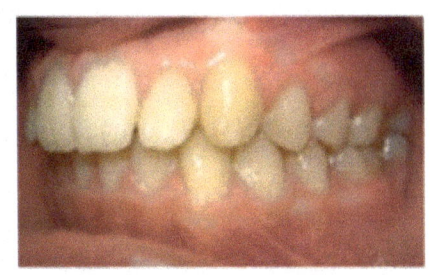

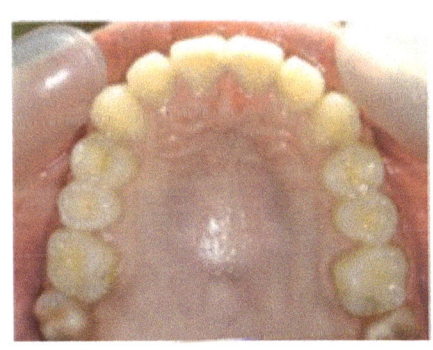 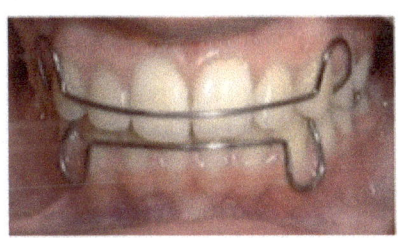 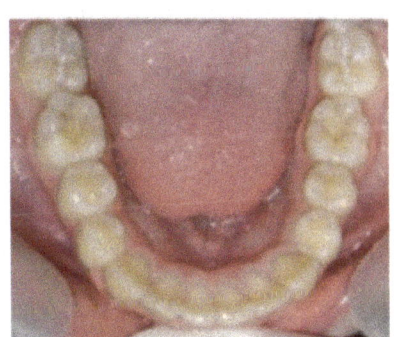

The patient is now aged 15 and is wearing upper and lower removable retainers Interdental stripping has been carried out to flatten the contacts between the lower anterior teeth. This is normally extended to the mesial of the first premolar on each side.

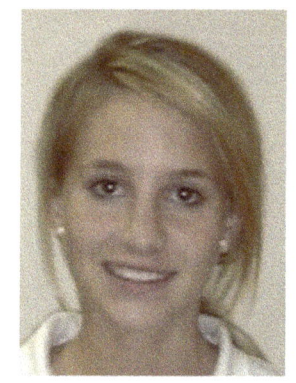
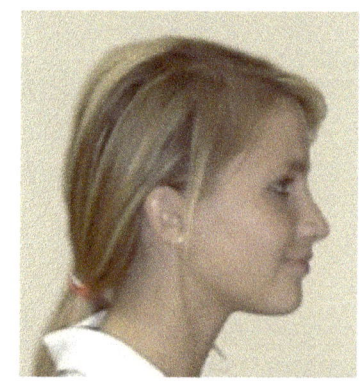
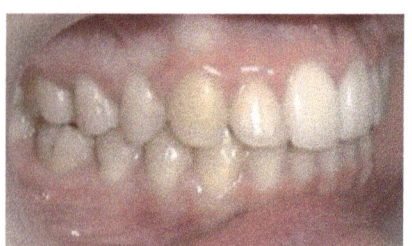
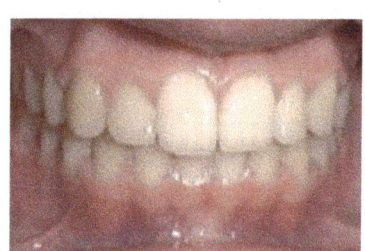
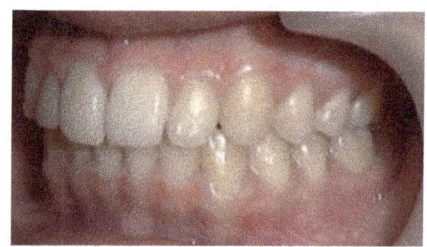
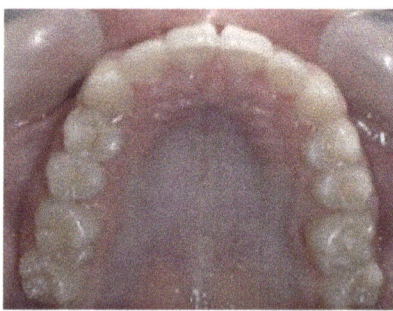
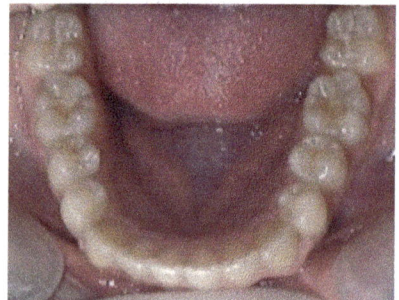

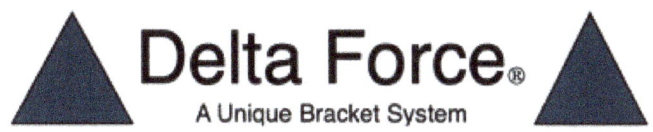

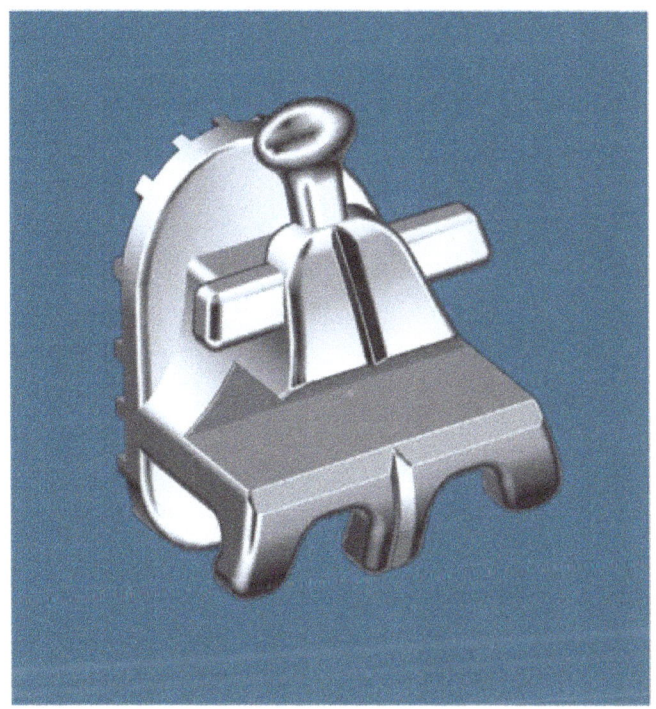

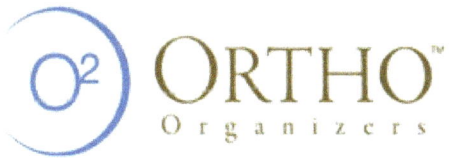

Unique Design

Easy Bracket Placement

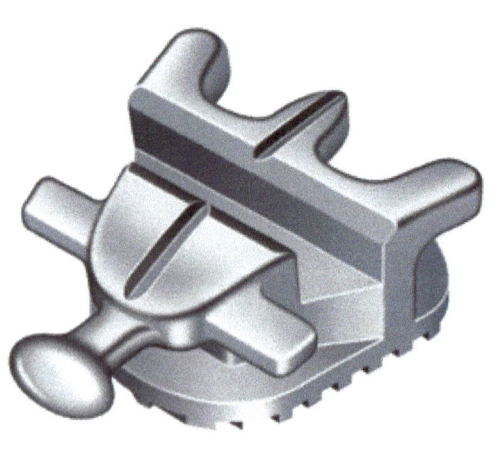

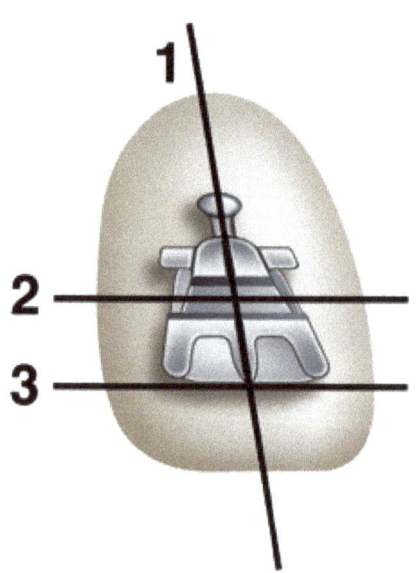

1

2

3

Crossbar gives additional control

Delta Force Bracket Tweezers

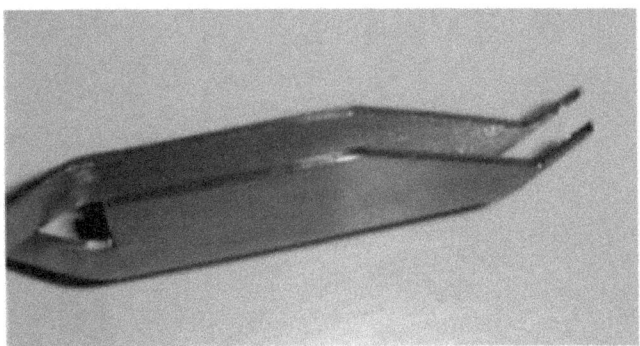

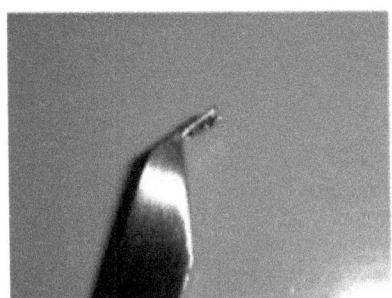
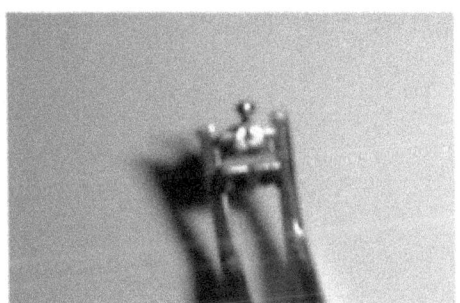

For Easy Bracket Placement

Bracket Width

Improves Archwire Deflection

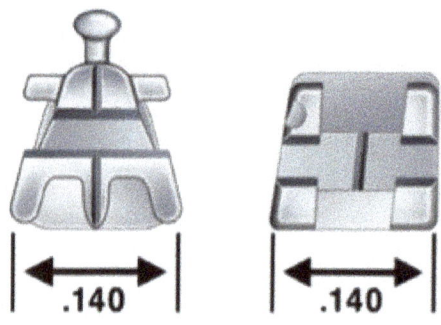

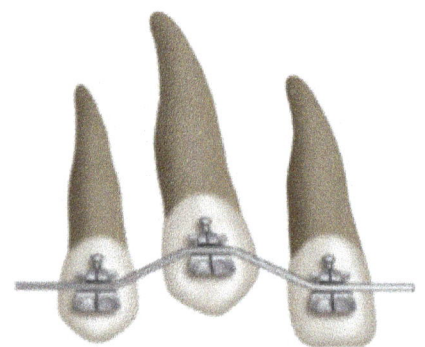

.140　　　.140

Increased Inter-Bracket Distance

Delta Force® is a registered trademark of Ortho Organizers

VARIABLE LIGATION OPTIONS

Minimal Friction

Medium Force

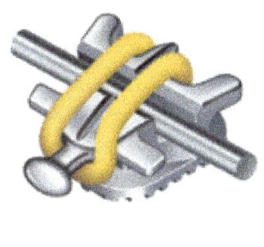
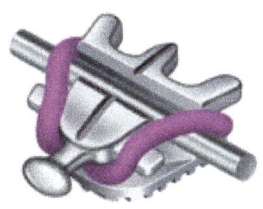

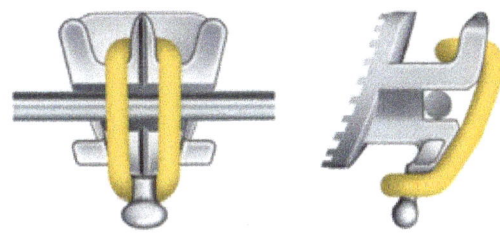
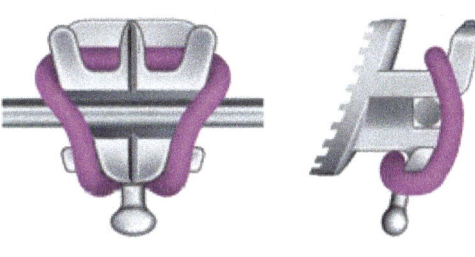

Free Sliding

Level & Align

Improved Finishing

Additional Force

Maximum Force

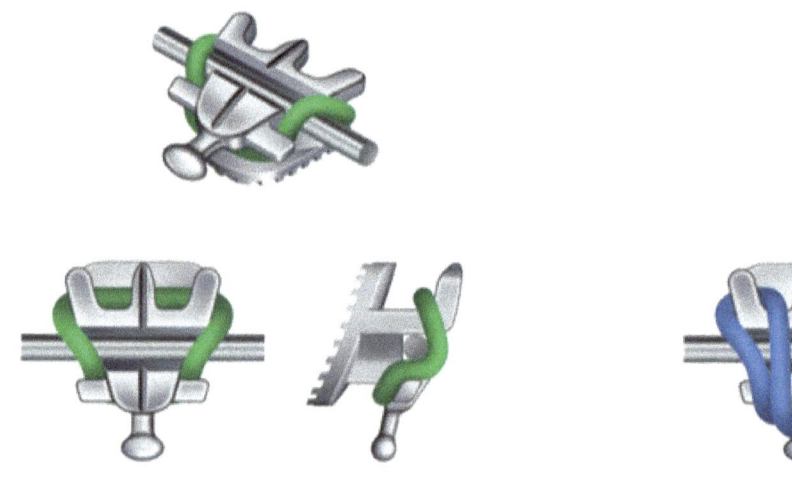

Finishing Ligation

Detailed Finishing

THE ROTATION WEDGE

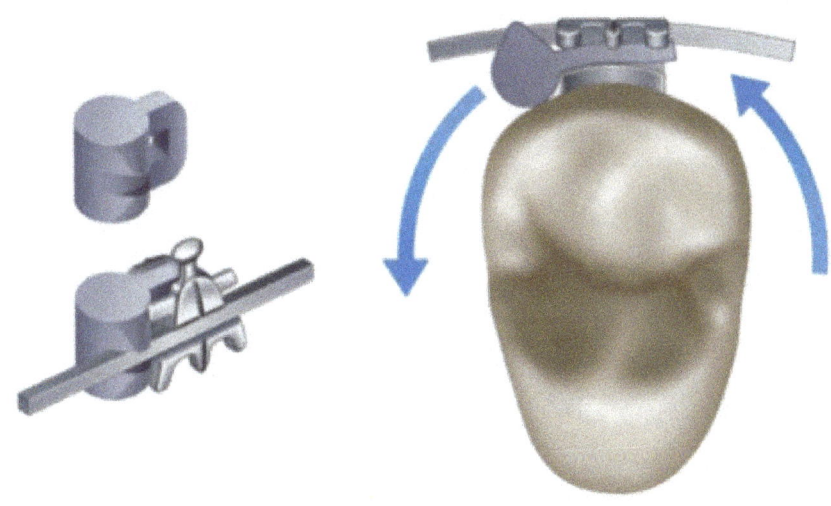

For Improved Control Of Severe Rotations

THE ROTATION TIE

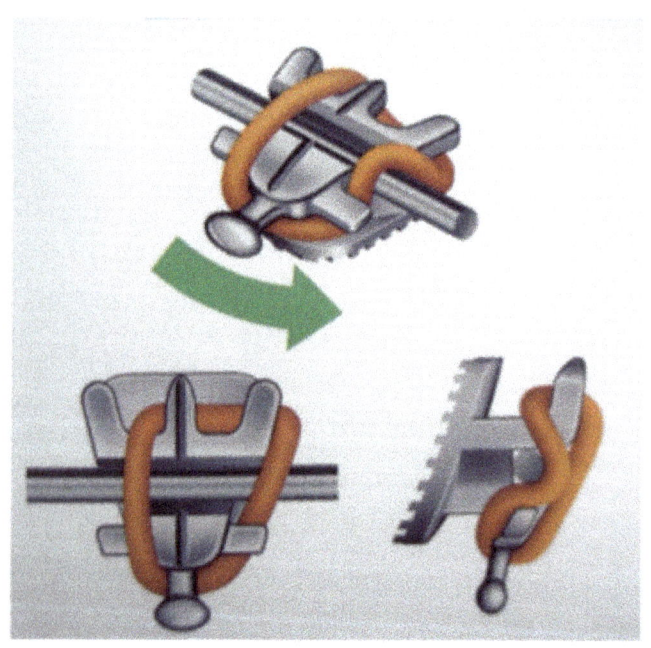

Extra rotation can be created by ligating behind one tie wing & under the crossbar on one side.

Rotation will occur towards the non ligated tie wing

Rapid movements with fewer appointments

IMPROVED TECHNOLOGY SHORTENS TREATMENT

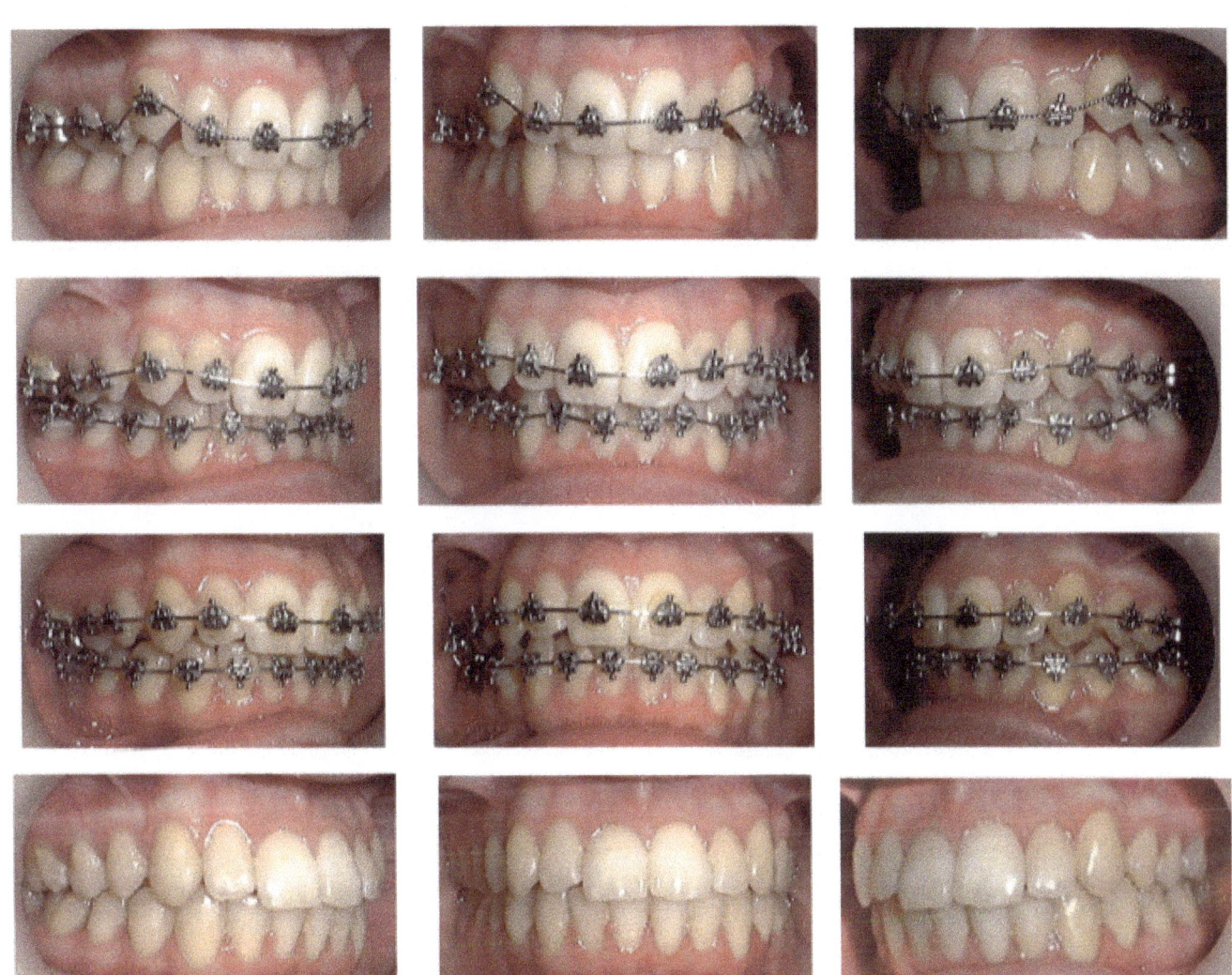

THE FORCE SYSTEM

TransForce Lingual Appliances & *Delta Force* Brackets
For superior control and enhanced treatment objectives

The first step in treatment in this case was maxillary expansion using the Transforce expander to correct a molar crossbite and develop the maxillary arch form. Light continuous forces applied by an enclosed nickel titanium spring in the TransForce appliance is an efficient mechanism to increase maxillary arch width. The crossbite was corrected within 3 months and the Transforce expander continued to expand for 4 months before fitting a fixed appliance.

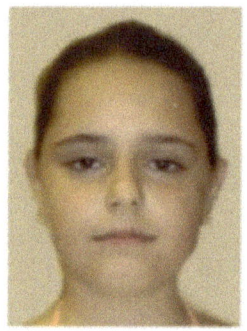 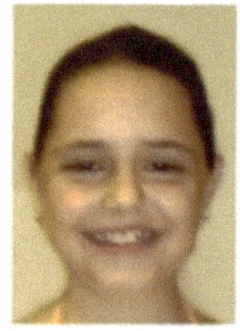 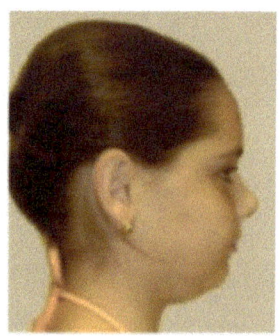

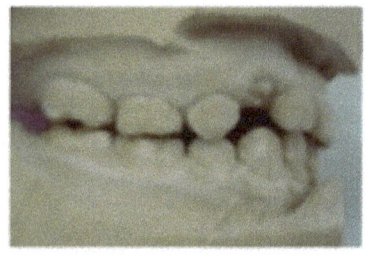 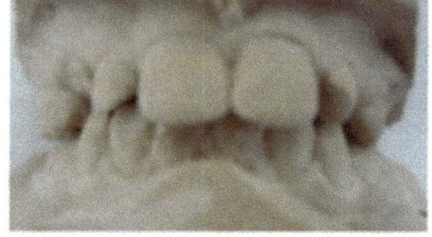 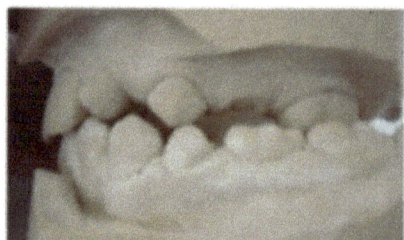

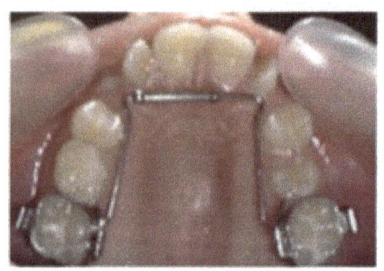 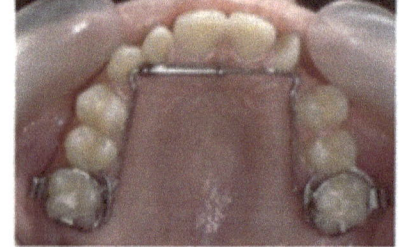 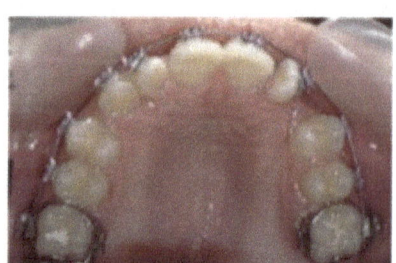

Further treatment was now required to correct anterior alignment and molar relationship and to make space for eruption of the crowded upper left canine. Delta Force brackets were selected for improved rotational control in correcting the severe rotation of an upper lateral incisor. The unique design of the Delta Force bracket is extremely effective in correcting severely displaced or rotated teeth. A significant mechanical advantage is achieved by the triangular shape with reduced width of the gingival tie wing combined with a gingival crossbar. This results in an increased inter-bracket distance and allows the archwire to flex into the bracket slot of severely displaced teeth. Control is improved at all stages of treatment by variable ligation to engage the wire progressively into the base of the bracket slot.

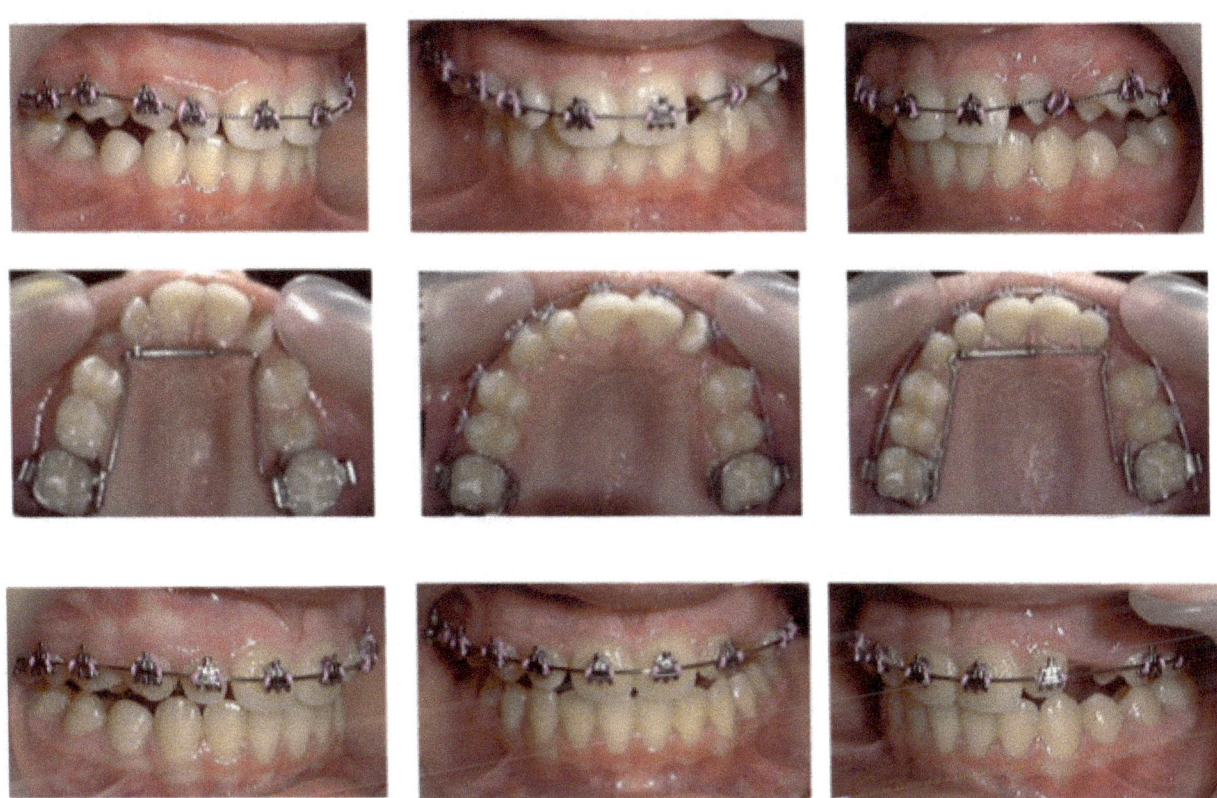

A Distalizing Arch was now fitted to make space to accommodate the unerupted canine and to correct the molar relationship. A lower lingual arch was fitted for anchorage with intermaxillary traction, conserving anchorage by the Elastic Load Reduction concept. Six ounces of elastic force is applied for 5 days, four ounces for 5 days and two ounces for 11 days before re-activating the coil springs and repeating the sequence. This method is designed for rapid movement of the molar, followed by repair and recovery. This physiological approach allows time for a logical sequence of cellular activity.

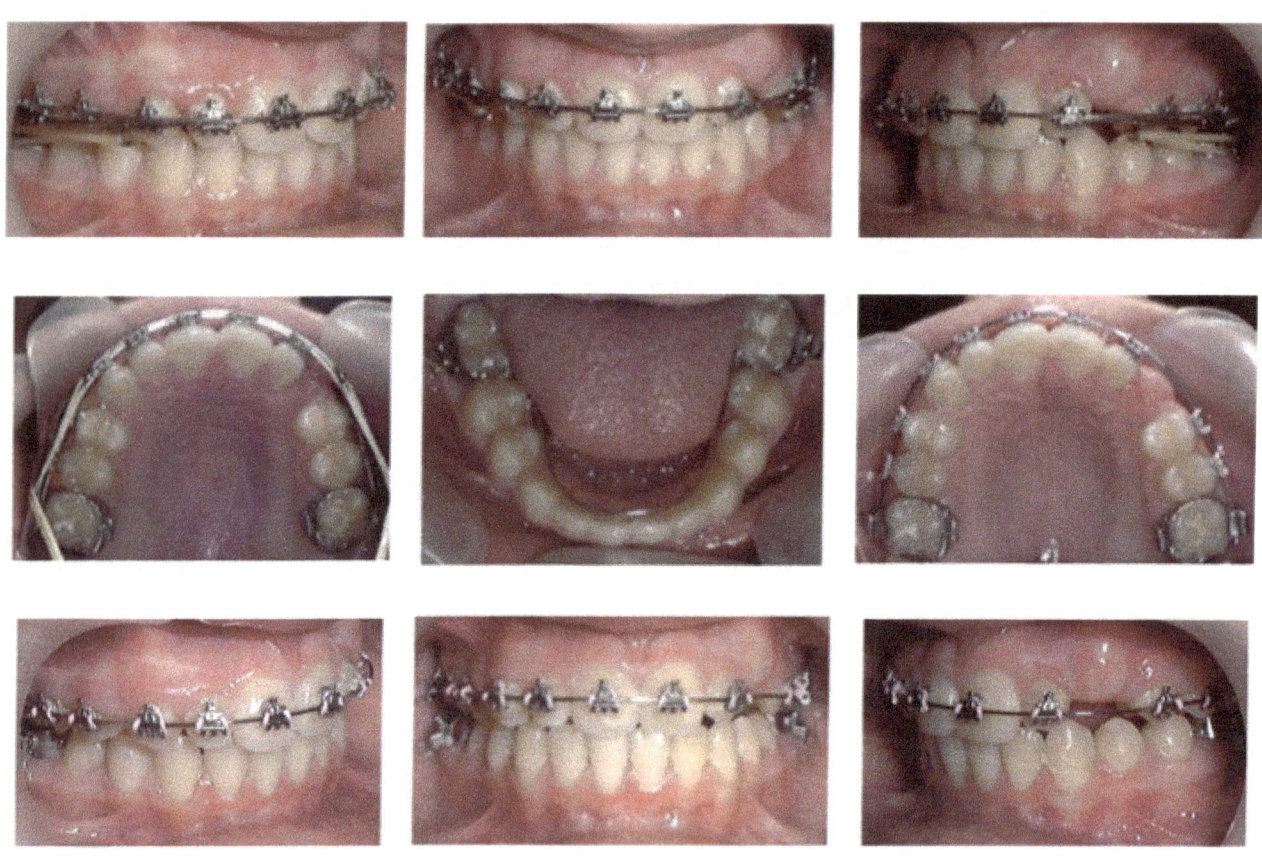

The Delta Force bracket allows early engagement of the archwire in the slot of the bracket when the canine erupts. A Delta force rotation wedge is applied to overcorrect the rotation of the lateral incisor

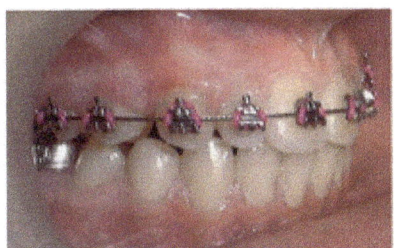
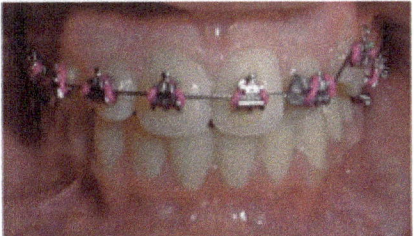
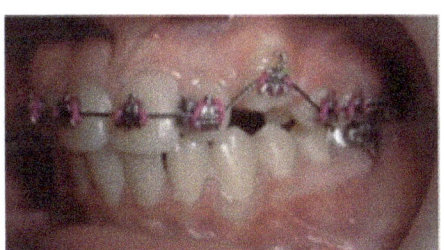

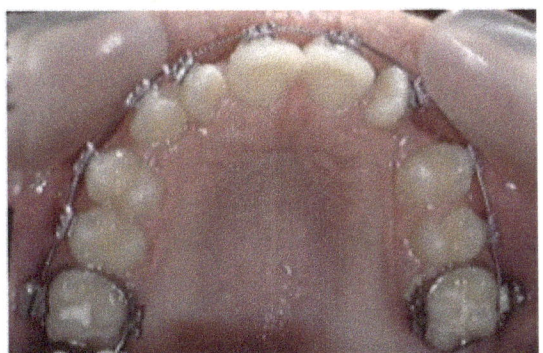
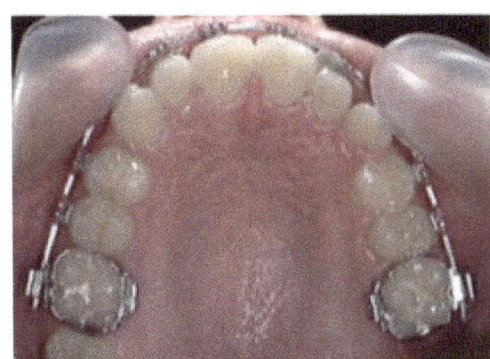

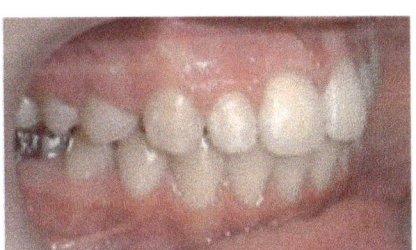
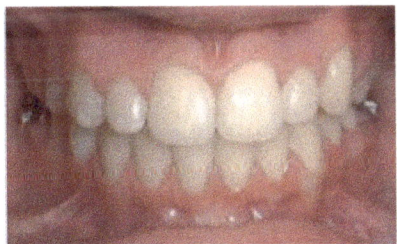
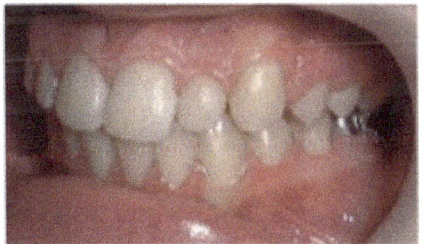

The Delta Force bracket allows early engagement of the archwire in the slot of the bracket when the canine erupts. A Delta force rotation wedge is applied to overcorrect the rotation of the lateral incisor

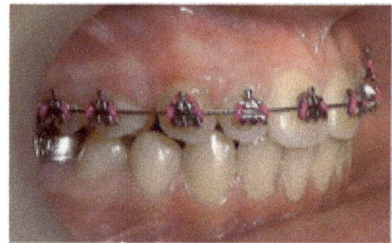
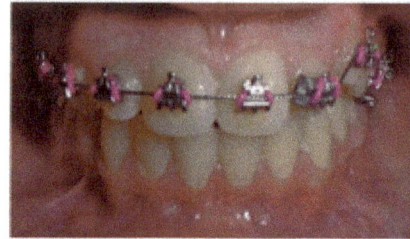
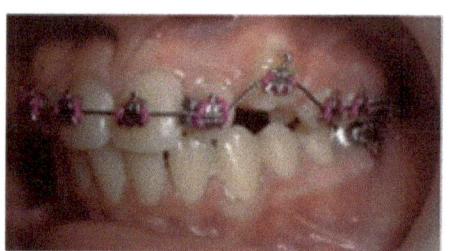

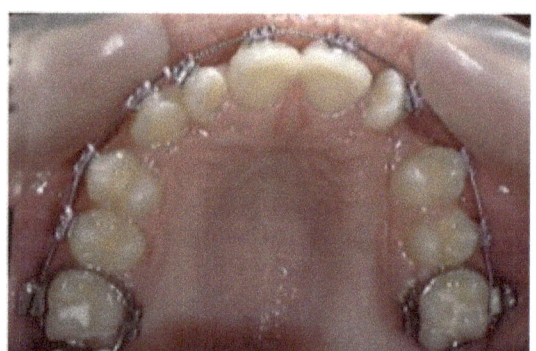
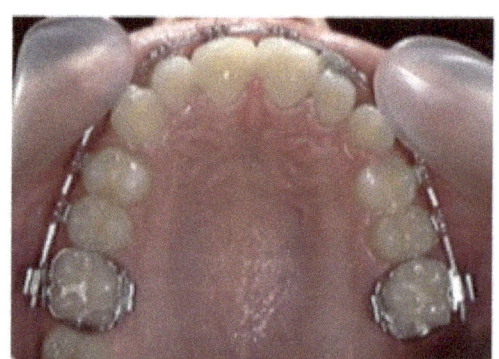

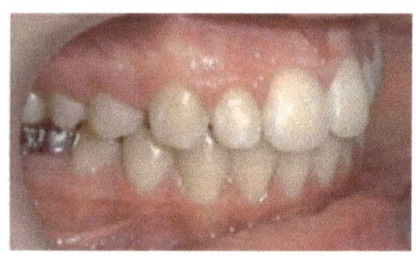
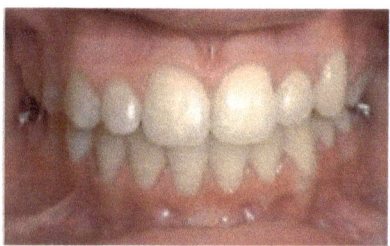
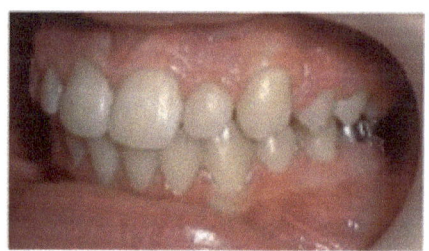

A Distalizing Arch was now fitted to make space to accommodate the unerupted canine and to correct the molar relationship. A lower lingual arch was fitted for anchorage with intermaxillary traction, conserving anchorage by the Elastic Load Reduction concept. Six ounces of elastic force is applied for 5 days, four ounces for 5 days and two ounces for 11 days before re-activating the coil springs and repeating the sequence. This method is designed for rapid movement of the molar, followed by repair and recovery. This physiological approach allows time for a logical sequence of cellular activity.

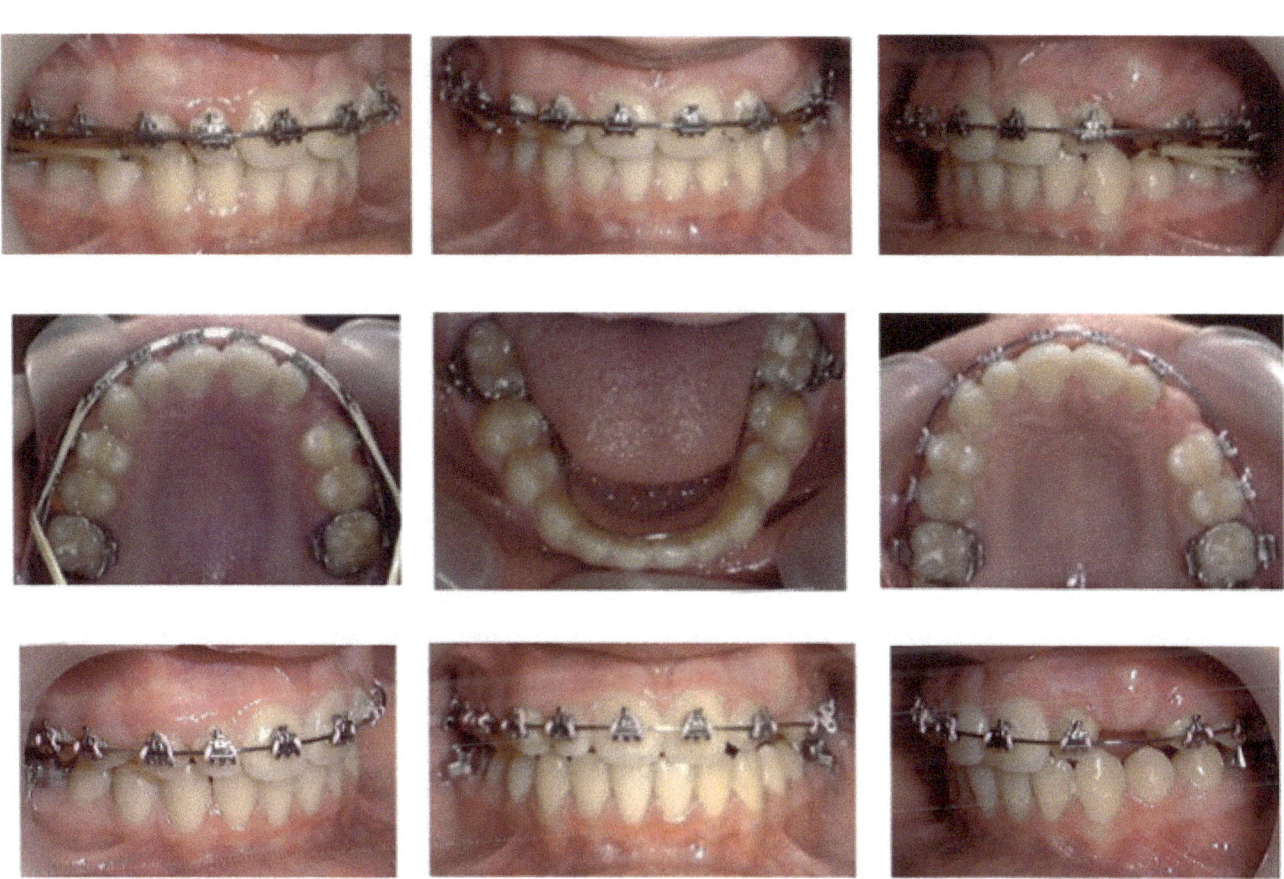

The Delta Force bracket allows early engagement of the archwire in the slot of the bracket when the canine erupts. A Delta force rotation wedge is applied to overcorrect the rotation of the lateral incisor

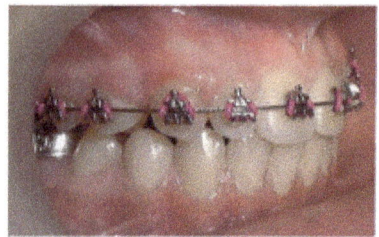
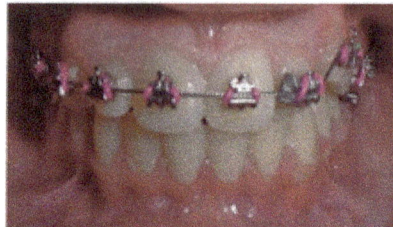
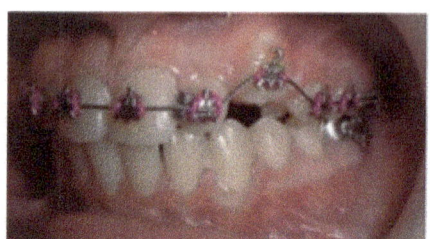

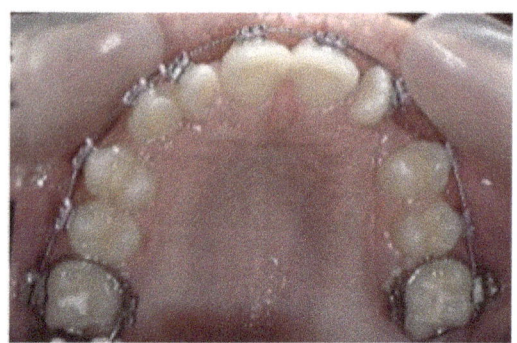
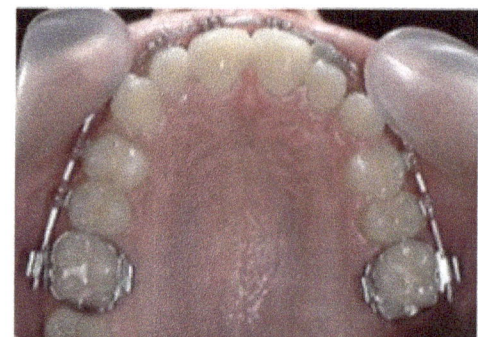

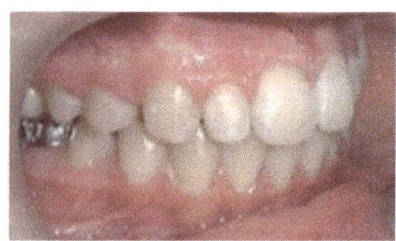
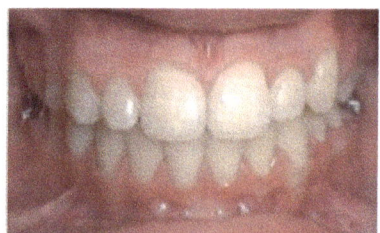
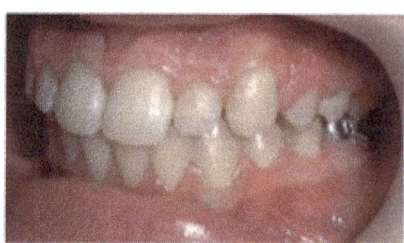

Active treatment was followed by one year with a removable retainer. Final records show the position one year out of retention at age 16. The severe rotation of the upper lateral incisor is corrected and stability of the occlusion and the rotated incisor is confirmed.

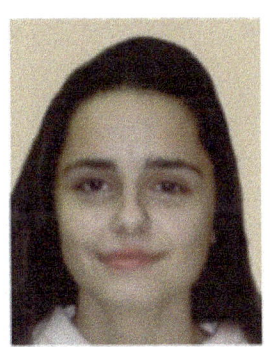
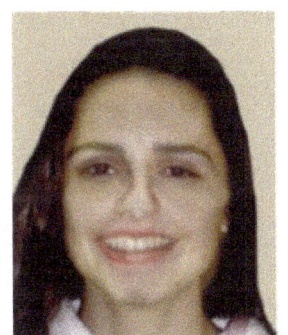
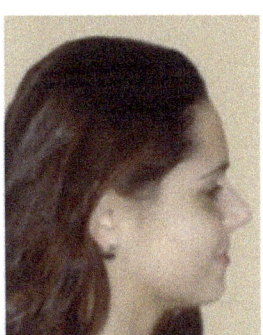

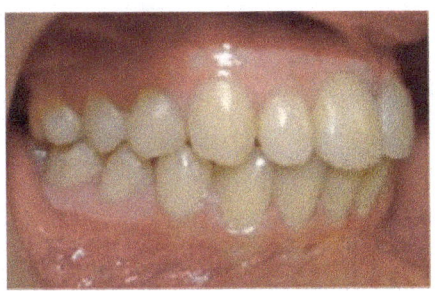
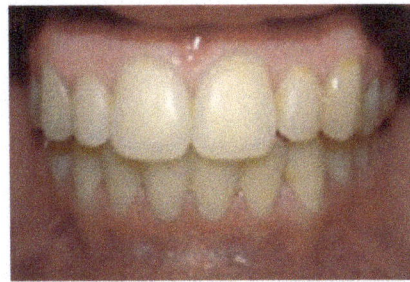
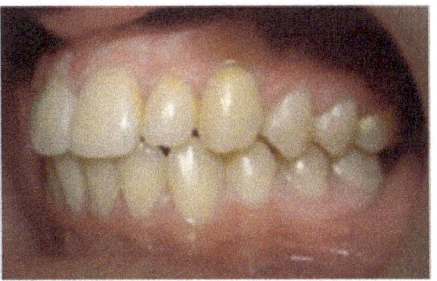

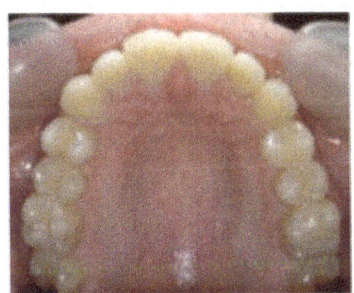
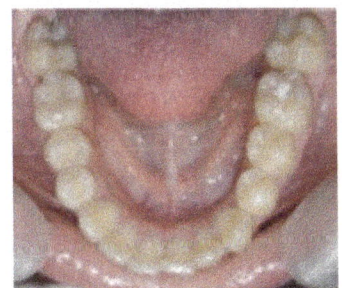

EXTRACTION THERAPY IN A DOLICHOFACIAL PATTERN

Extraction therapy is necessary to resolve crowding in this delicate dolichofacial pattern. Braces can be a fashion accessory, as this young girl demonstrates! She is very happy to smile and show off her new fixed appliance, which matches her jewellery perfectly. The most important decision during the appointment is 'What colour of elastics shall we choose today?' This is especially important for young ladies of all ages!

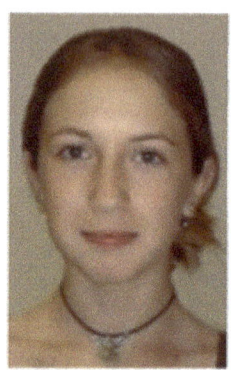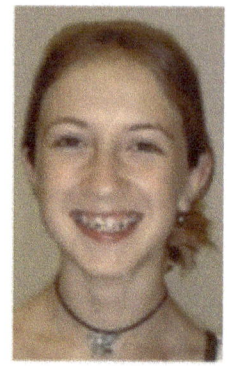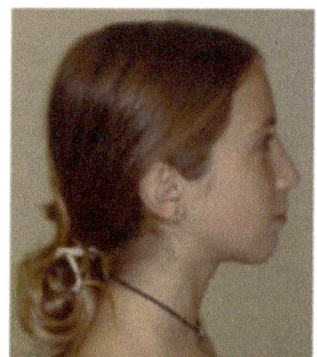

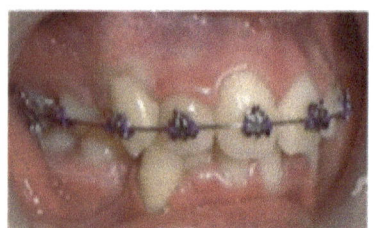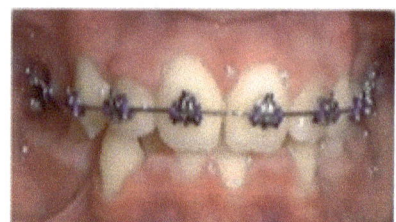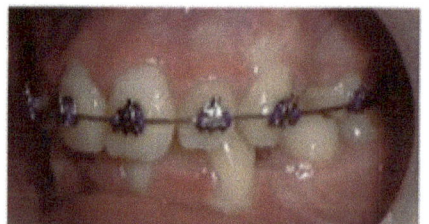

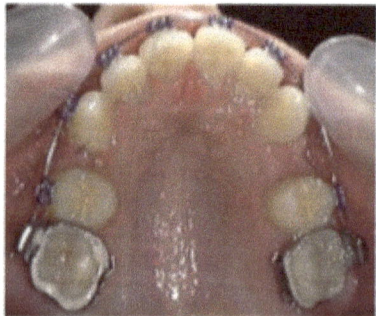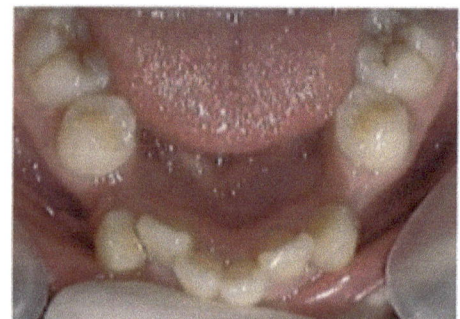

When the lower appliance is fitted we have a wider choice of colours. For this bright young lady it would be boring to have the same colour in both arches. The bright pink is sure to draw attention combined with a subdued black in the lower. Occlusal views show excellent progress at the next appointment in 10 weeks. Bite guides are fitted to prevent damage to the lower appliance.

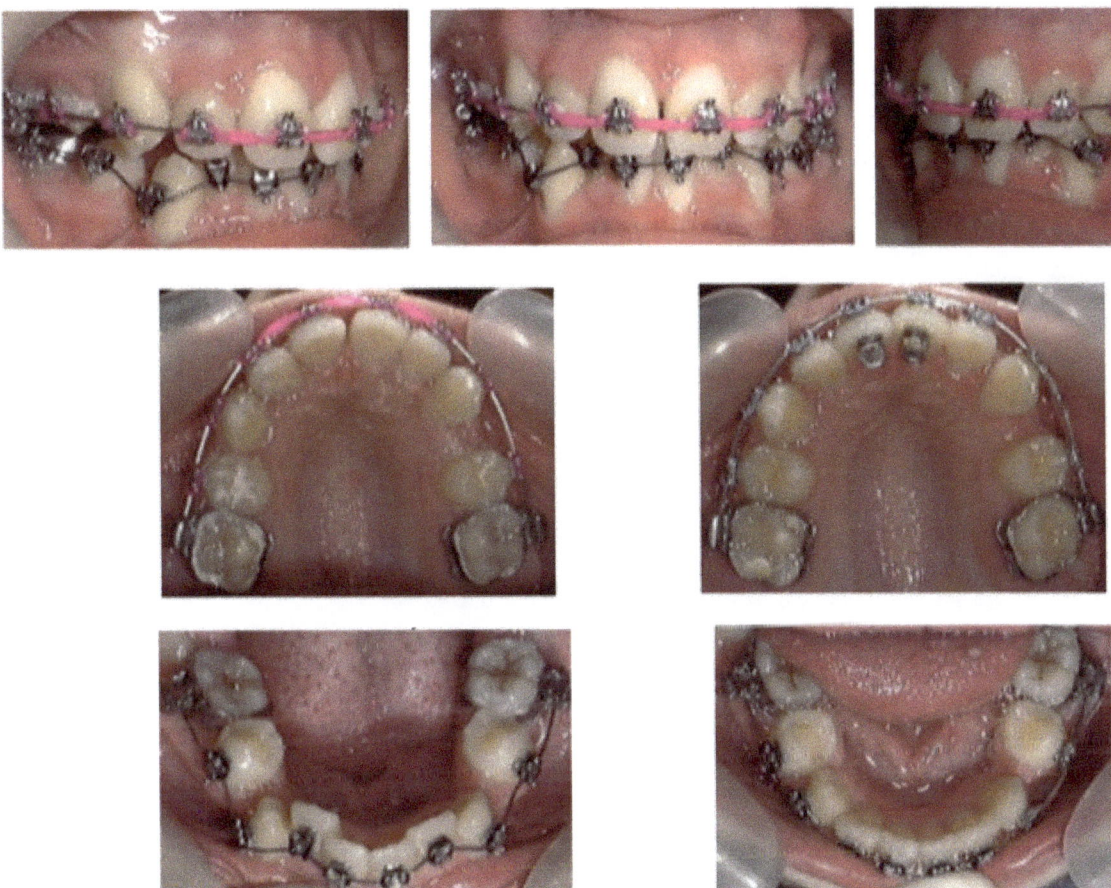

Today, after much deliberation, we go for pastel colours with pale pink in the upper and violet in the lower. The pale pink proved so popular that it is retained at the next visit and back to black for the lower. Treatment is proceeding well and spaces are closing nicely with power chain and the bite guides have helped to control the vertical and reduce the overbite.

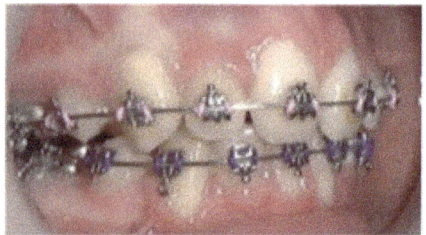
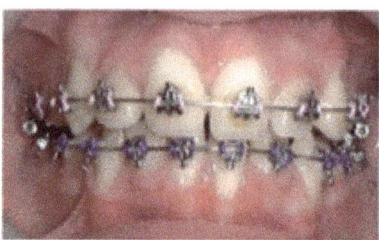
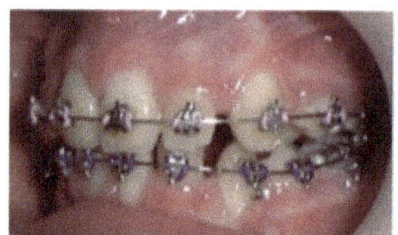

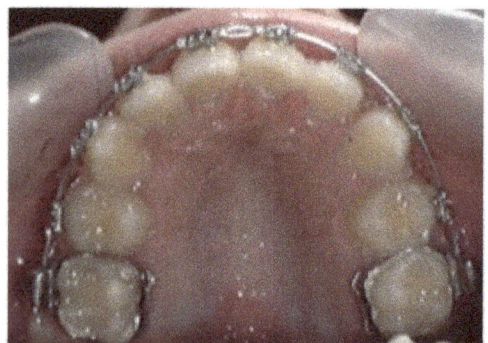
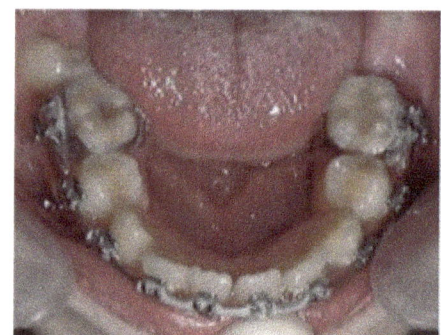

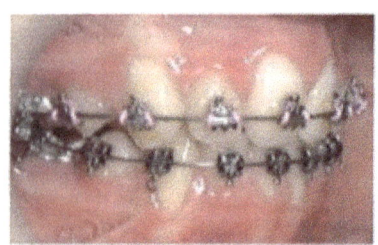
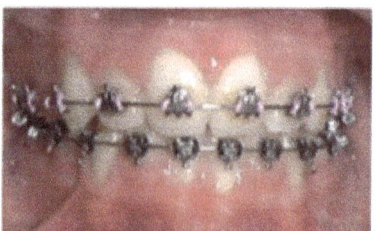
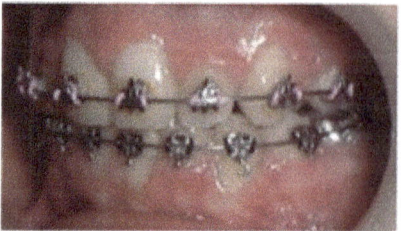

Treatment was completed in 20 months and 10 appointments. The day we remove the braces Sara cannot stop smiling! It is always a red letter day in the life of a young patient when they see the result of their good cooperation. At the end of the day it was worth it! The reward is a beautiful smile for the rest of your life.

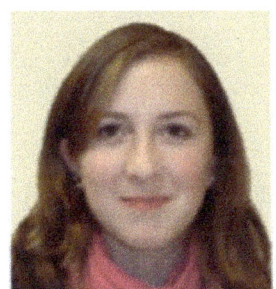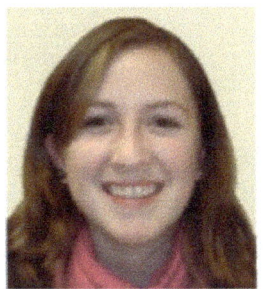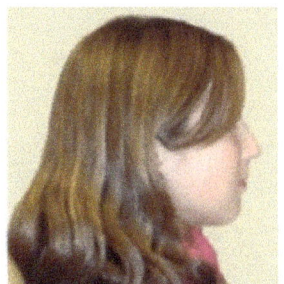

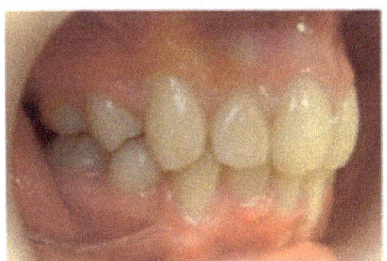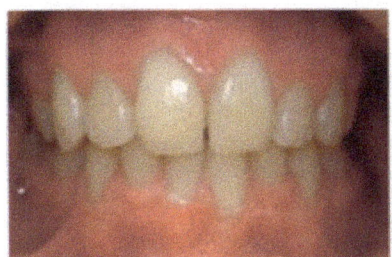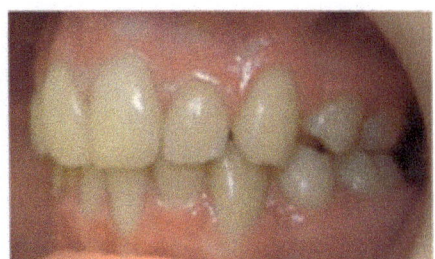

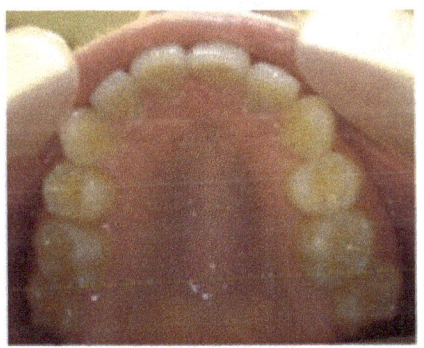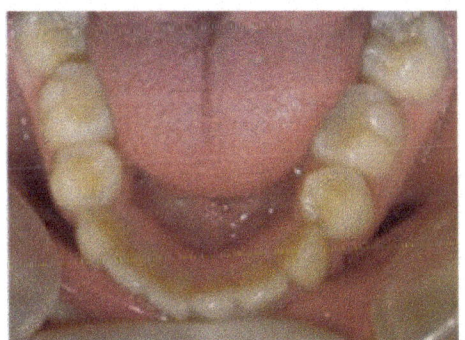

Cranial Base Angle 27°: Facial Axis 24°: Mandibular Plane 33° Convexity 8 mm

The dolichofacial pattern is confirmed by increased mandibular plane angle and cranio-mandibular angle, while the facial axis angle is reduced. The convexity is 8 mm, although the buccal segment relationship is Class I. The lower incisors are 4 mm ahead of the A-Po line and these factors combined with lower labial and distal crowding were the basis for premolar extractions. This approach is reflected in the end result as the profile is flatter after treatment

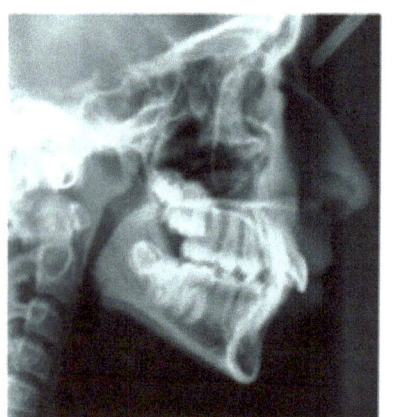
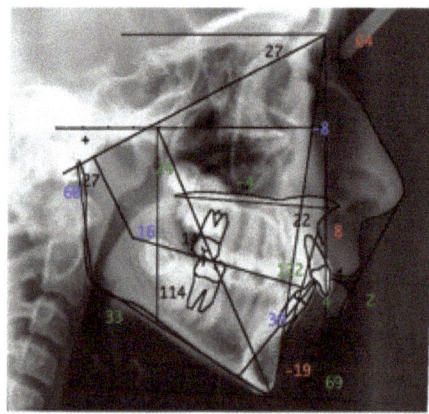
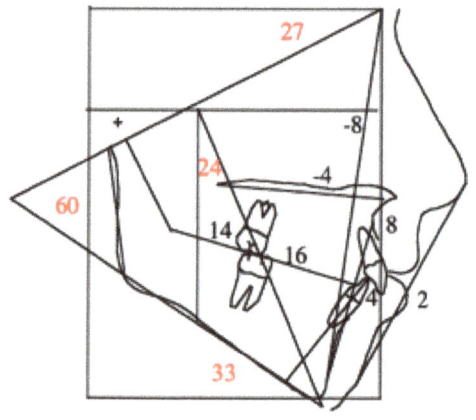

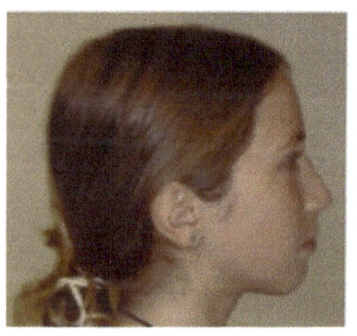
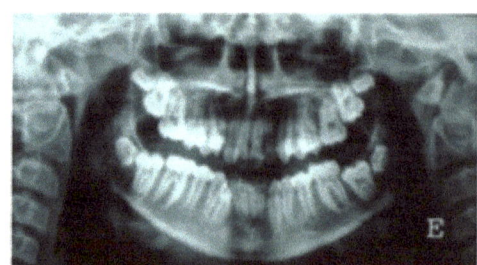
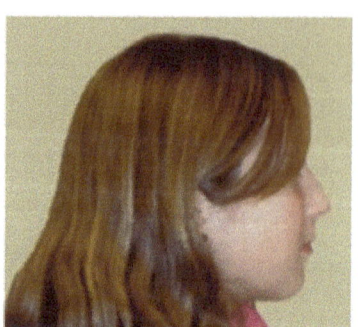

EXTRACTION THERAPY IN A SEVERE CLASS II DIVISION I MALOCCLUSION

This girl has a severe Class II Division I malocclusion with an anterior open bite and lower arch crowding The original treatment plan was to use fixed appliances in the first stage to resolve crowding and align the arches. followed by functional therapy with Twin Blocks to advance the mandible and correct the distal occlusion. A lower fixed appliance was fitted first

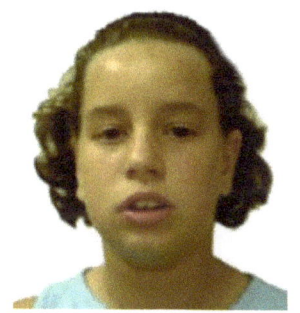 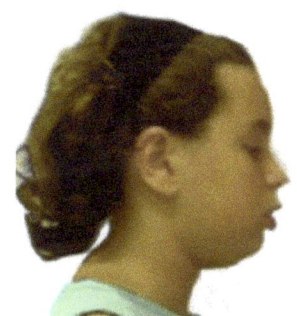

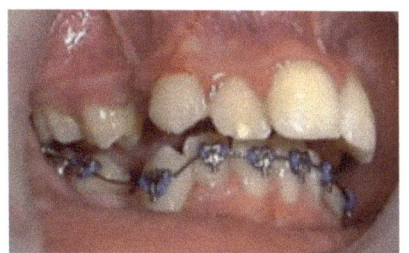 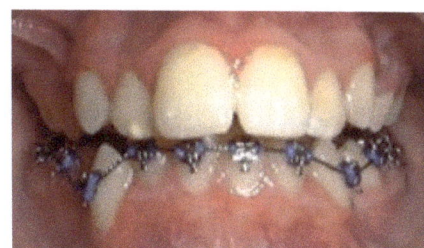 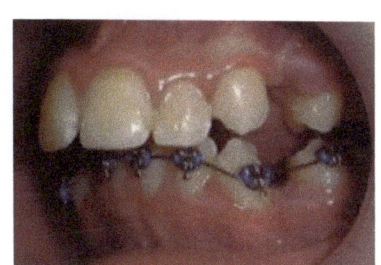

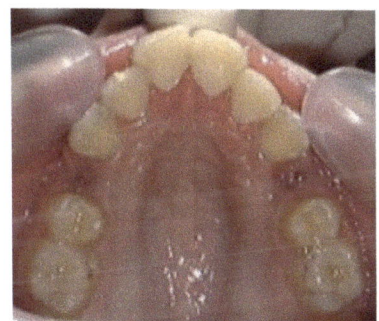 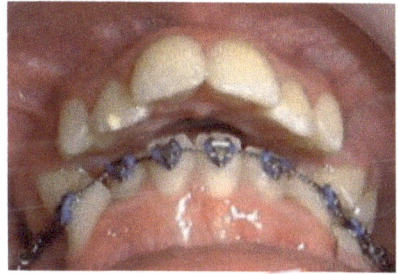 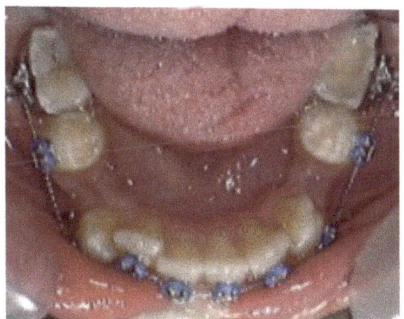

After the initial stage of space closure the patient moved away to Lisbon in the middle of treatment, and was not easily accessible for appointments, so the treatment plan was simplified to complete the treatment with fixed appliances and Class II mechanics. This was successful in reducing the overjet and overbite and improving the distal occlusion for orthodontic correction.

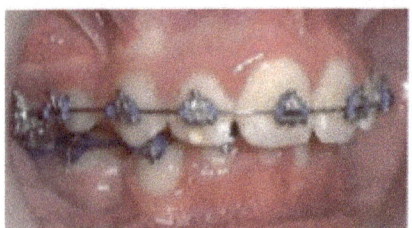
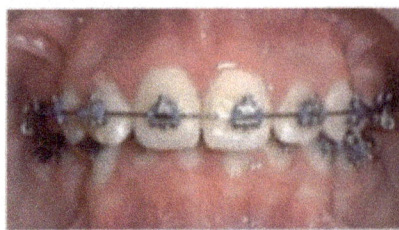
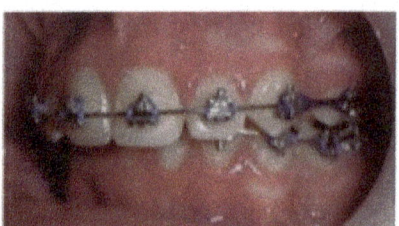

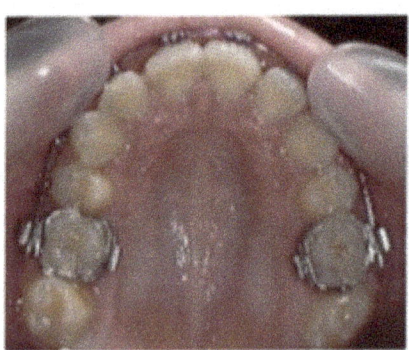
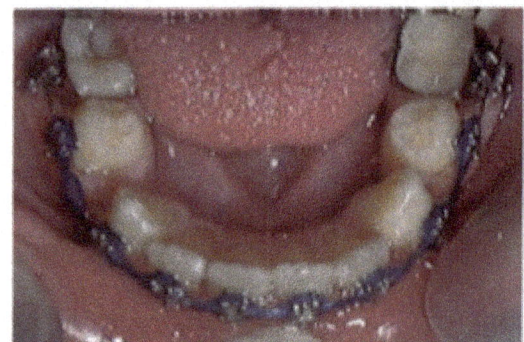

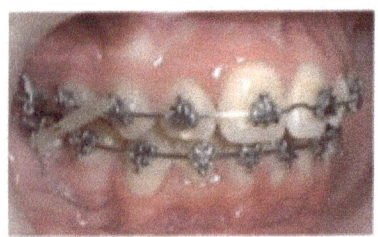
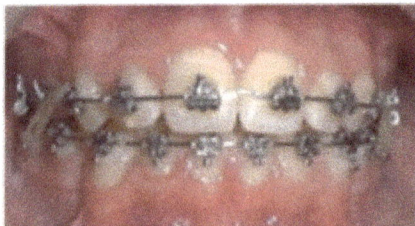
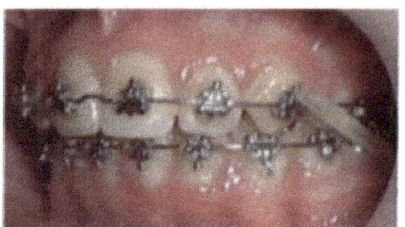

The limitation in this approach is that it does not address the underlying skeletal problem and there must be a compromise in the facial changes that can be achieved. Correction by inter-maxillary elastic traction uses low forces to move the teeth and treatment takes significantly longer to complete compared to functional therapy to advance the mandible.

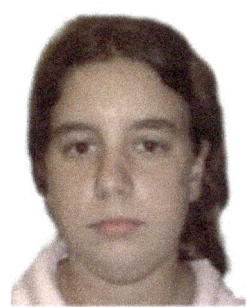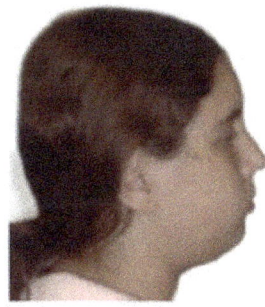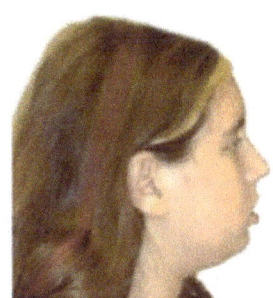

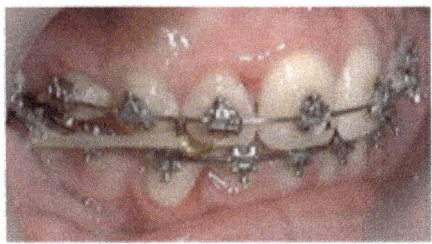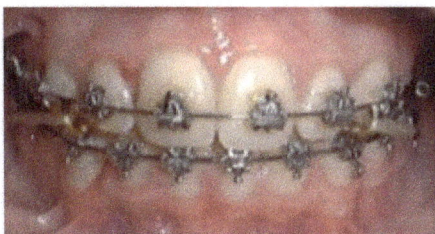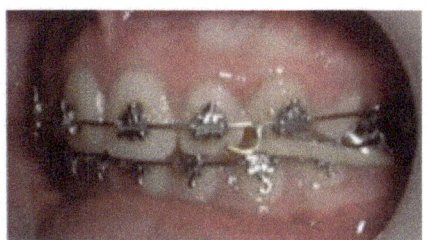

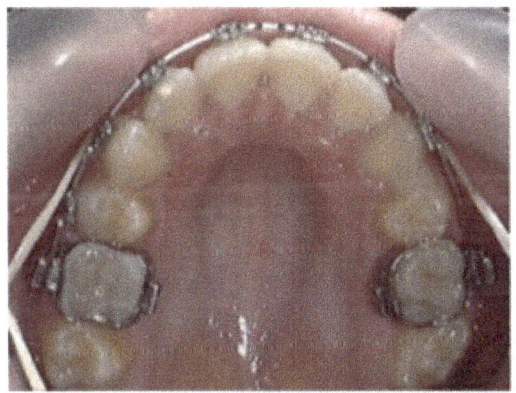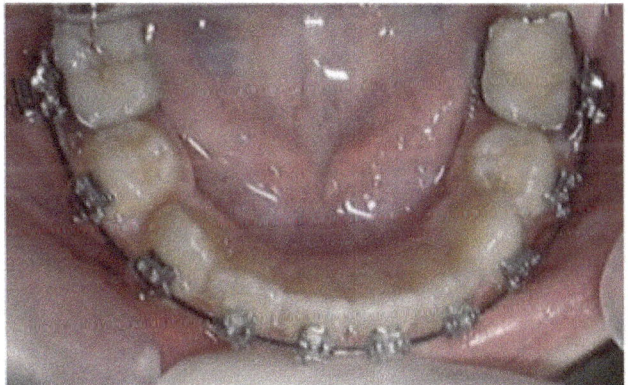

Final records show the position after 3 years treatment and retention continued for a year with removable retainers. After treatment there was still a tendency to adopt an incompetent lip posture, as shown on the previous page and the skeletal Class II pattern was still evident.

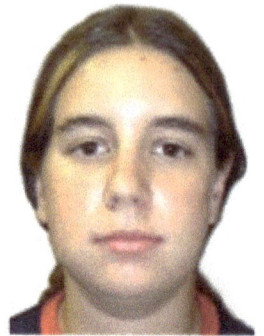
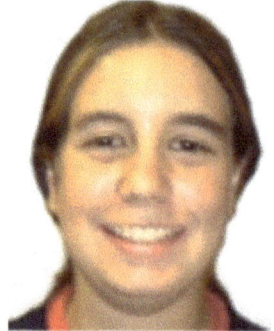
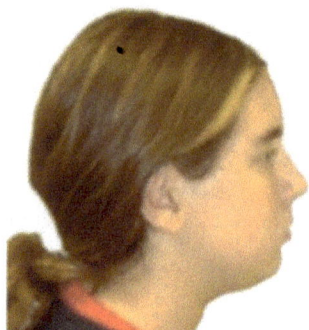

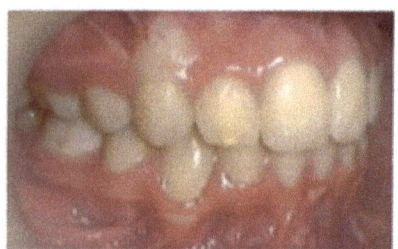
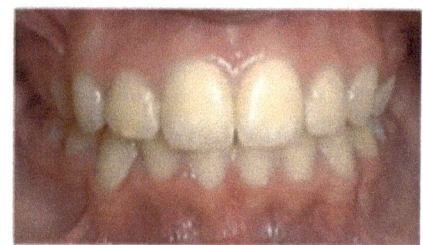
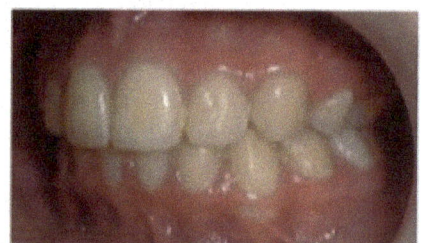

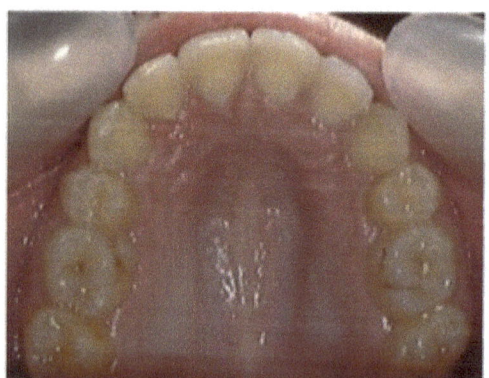
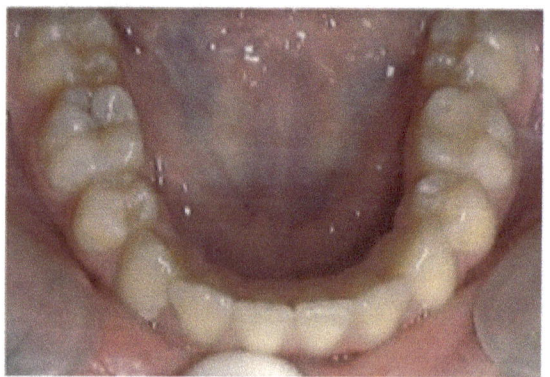

Cranial Base Angle 28°: Facial Axis 25°: Mandibular Plane 30° Convexity 9 mm

Cephalometric analysis confirmed a severe Class II skeletal base relationship with 9 mm convexity with an increased mandibular plane angle and increased lower facial height. The panoramic radiograph showed potential crowding of third molars. An alternative approach might have been extraction of second molars and a bioprogressive approach as the lower incisors were lingual to the A-Po line. A functional component could have improved the class II skeletal pattern.

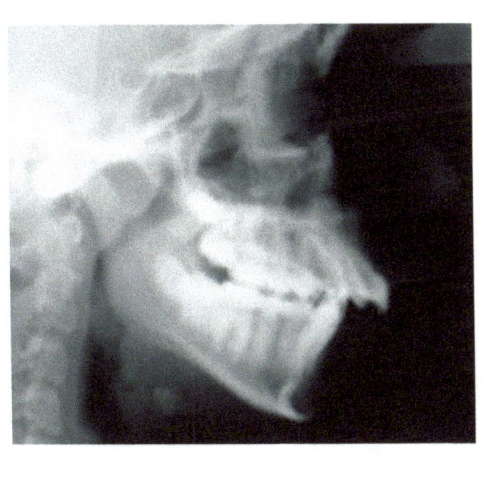
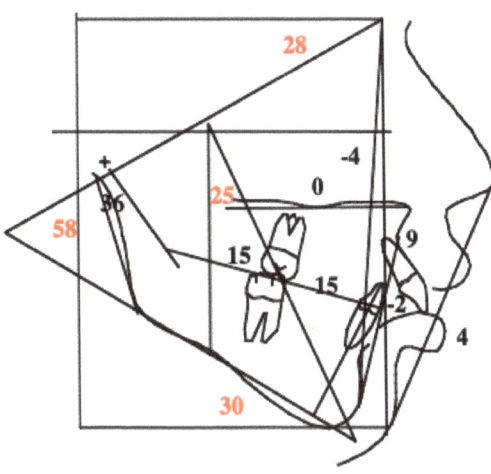

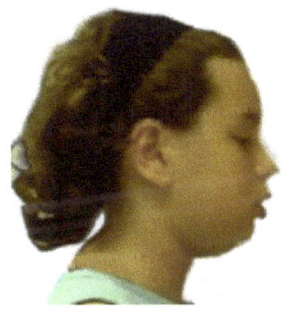
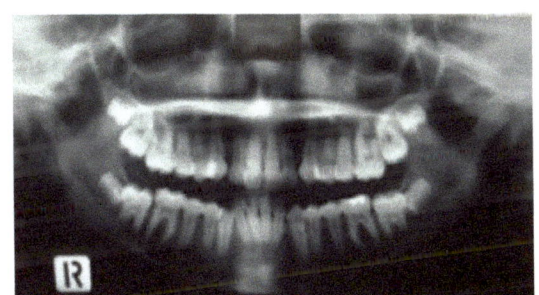
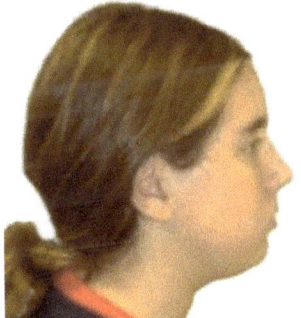

FIXED TWIN BLOCKS IN SEVERE DOLICHOFACIAL PATTERN

This young girl presents a Class II Division I malocclusion with severe maxillary contraction, resulting in anterior crowding. Upper lateral incisors are severely rotated. An anterior open bite tendency is related to tongue thrust and the underlying skeletal pattern is severe dolichofacial.

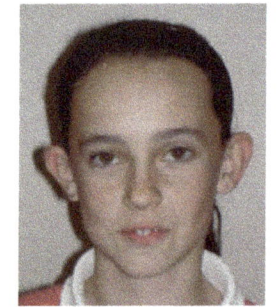
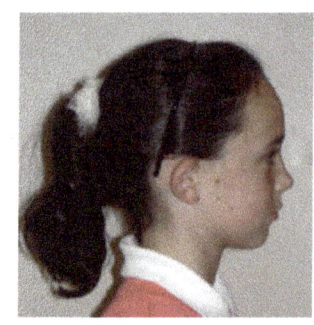

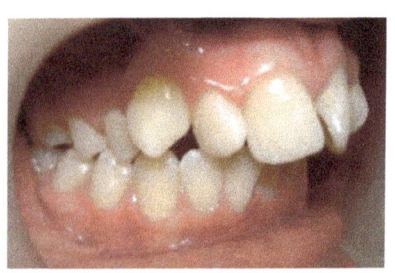
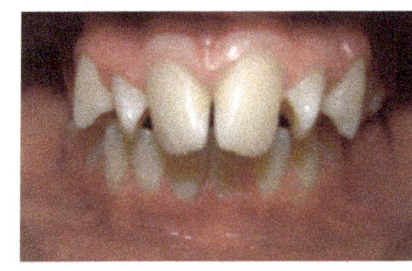
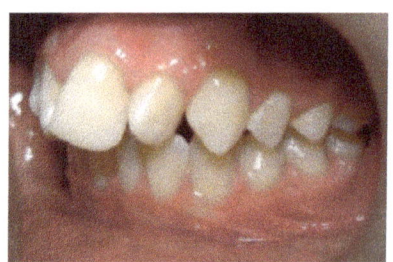

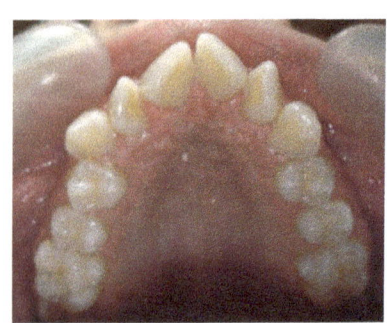
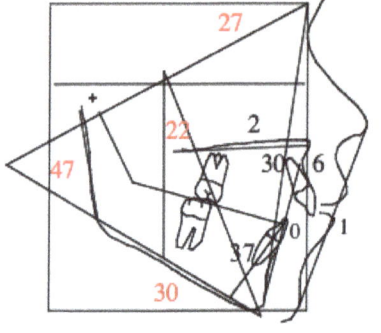
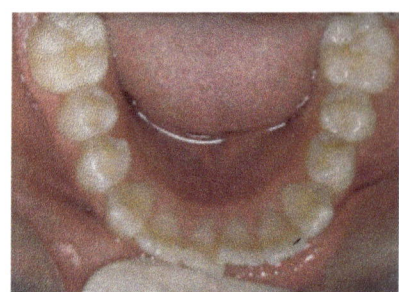

Before Treatment: Cranial Base Angle 27 °: Facial Axis 22 °: Mandibular Plane 30 ° Convexity 6 mm

EXCELLENT ROTATIONAL CONTROL & ARCH DEVELOPMENT

TransForce lingual appliances initiate treatment for arch development to accommodate crowded upper anterior teeth. Delta Force brackets are fitted at the next visit to correct the severely rotated upper incisors. This combination of mechanics is very effective in creating space to align the teeth and controlling a difficult malocclusion. Children like colours and for that reason I normally use conventional bracket systems so that they can choose colours at each visit.

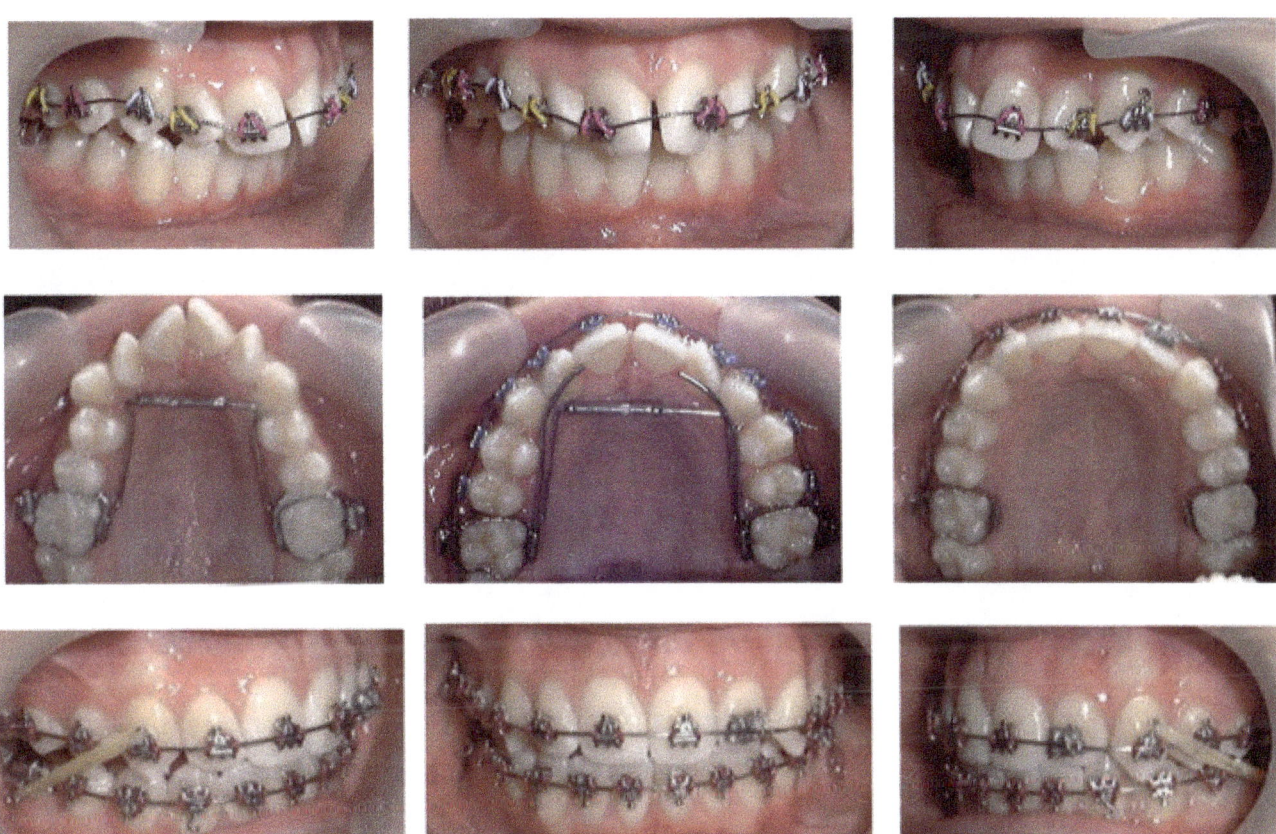

Maxillary expansion is an essential factor in treatment and an upper TransForce Transverse expansion appliance is fitted first, followed by an upper fixed appliance. Arch development creates space to align the anterior teeth in combination with the fixed appliance. Favourable effects on the facial contours by maxillary arch development are evident after 8 months treatment.

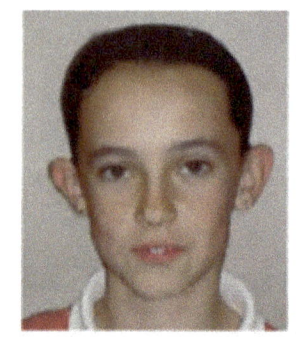 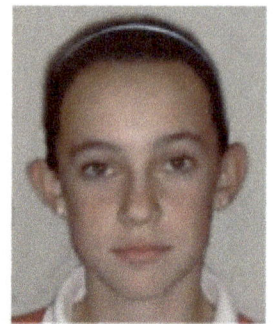

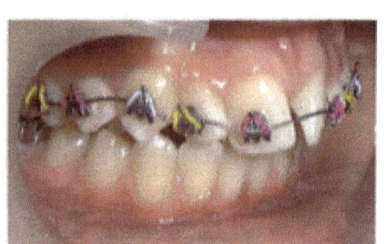 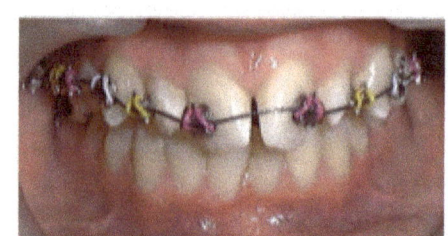 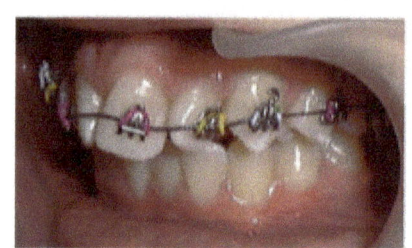

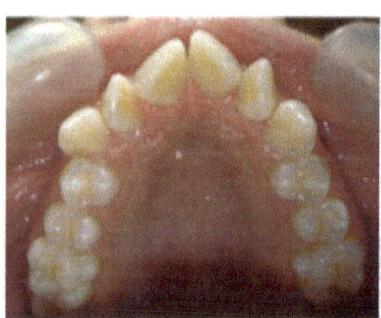 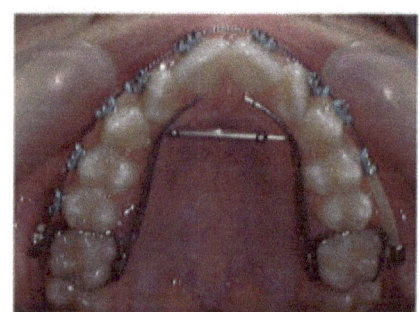 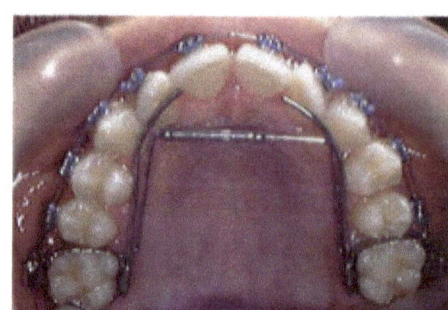

Significant problems remain of a severe anterior open bite and full unit distal occlusion. At this stage mandibular advancement is required to correct the distal occlusion and improve the profile. Fixed Twin Blocks are bonded directly to the teeth and power chain is extended to buccal buttons on the blocks for additional bucco-lingual stability. The addition of vertical box elastics worn at night is an important factor in closing the anterior open bite by applying intrusive forces to the posterior teeth.

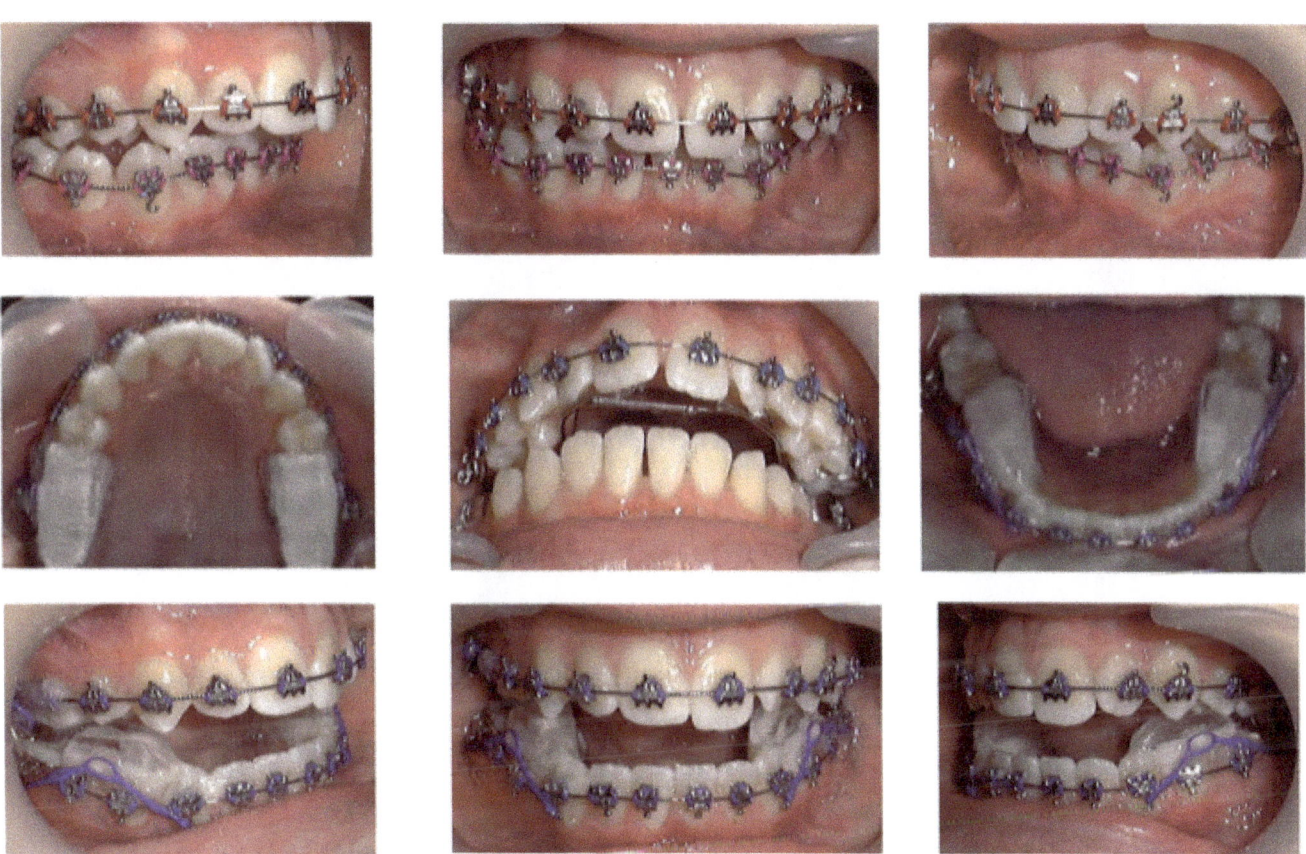

The Fixed Twin Blocks were removed after 6 months, when the distal occlusion is corrected and the profile has improved significantly. Further treatment is required to detail the occlusion with fixed appliances.

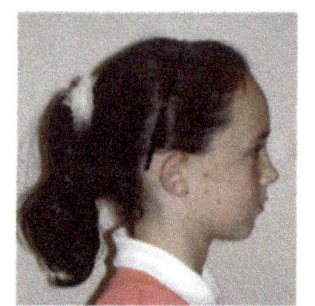 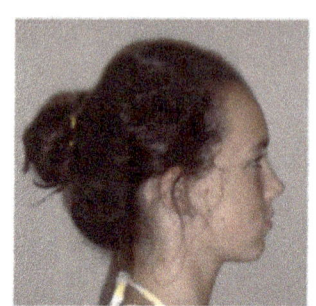

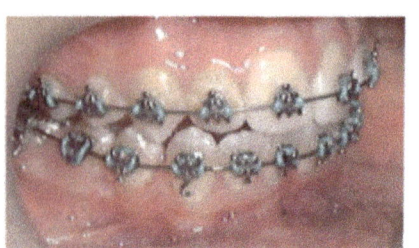 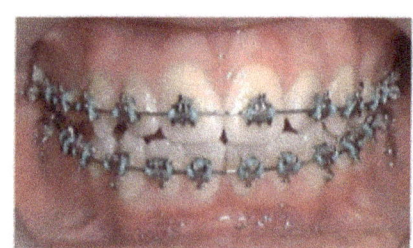 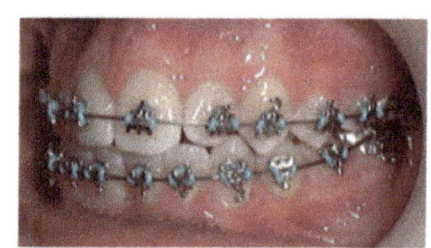

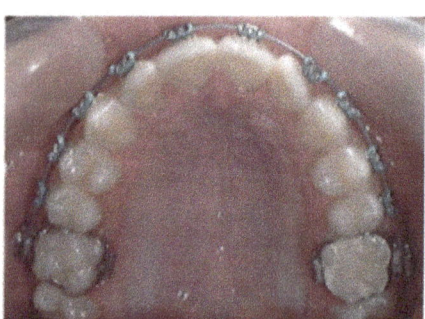 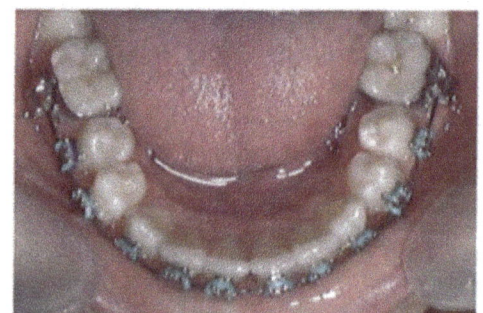

Profile photographs show the progress at this stage. In the middle photograph the mandible is postured forward to anticipate the expected change in the profile after treatment. This is a preview of the expected result. Fixed appliance treatment is continuing in this case as a rotation wedge improves the rotated incisor. At this stage the patient moved from Portugal to England. No completed records are available.

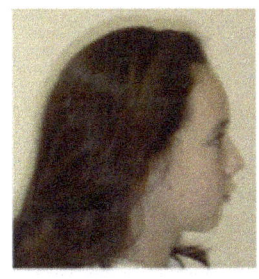 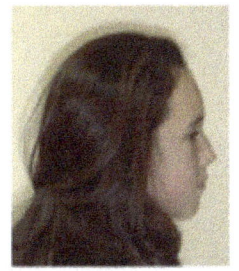 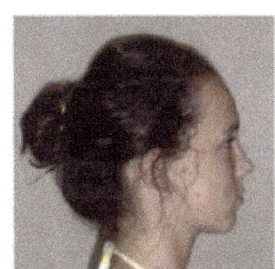

Before treatment Mandible Postured Forward After Twin Blocks

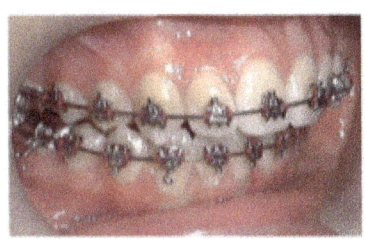 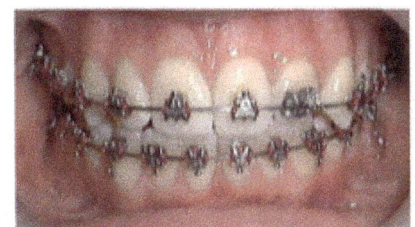 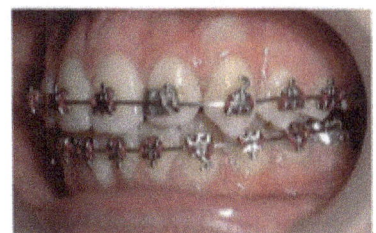

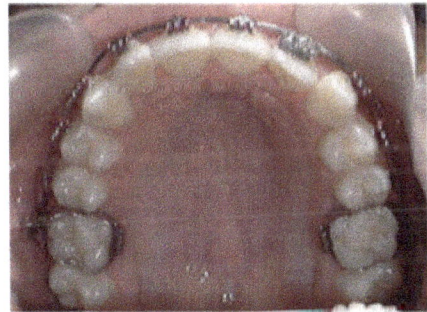 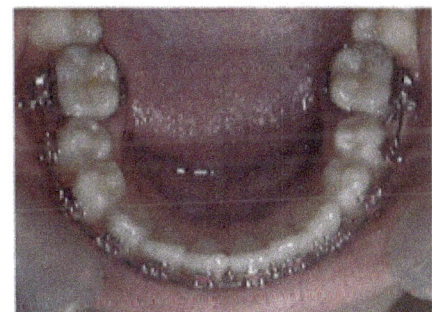

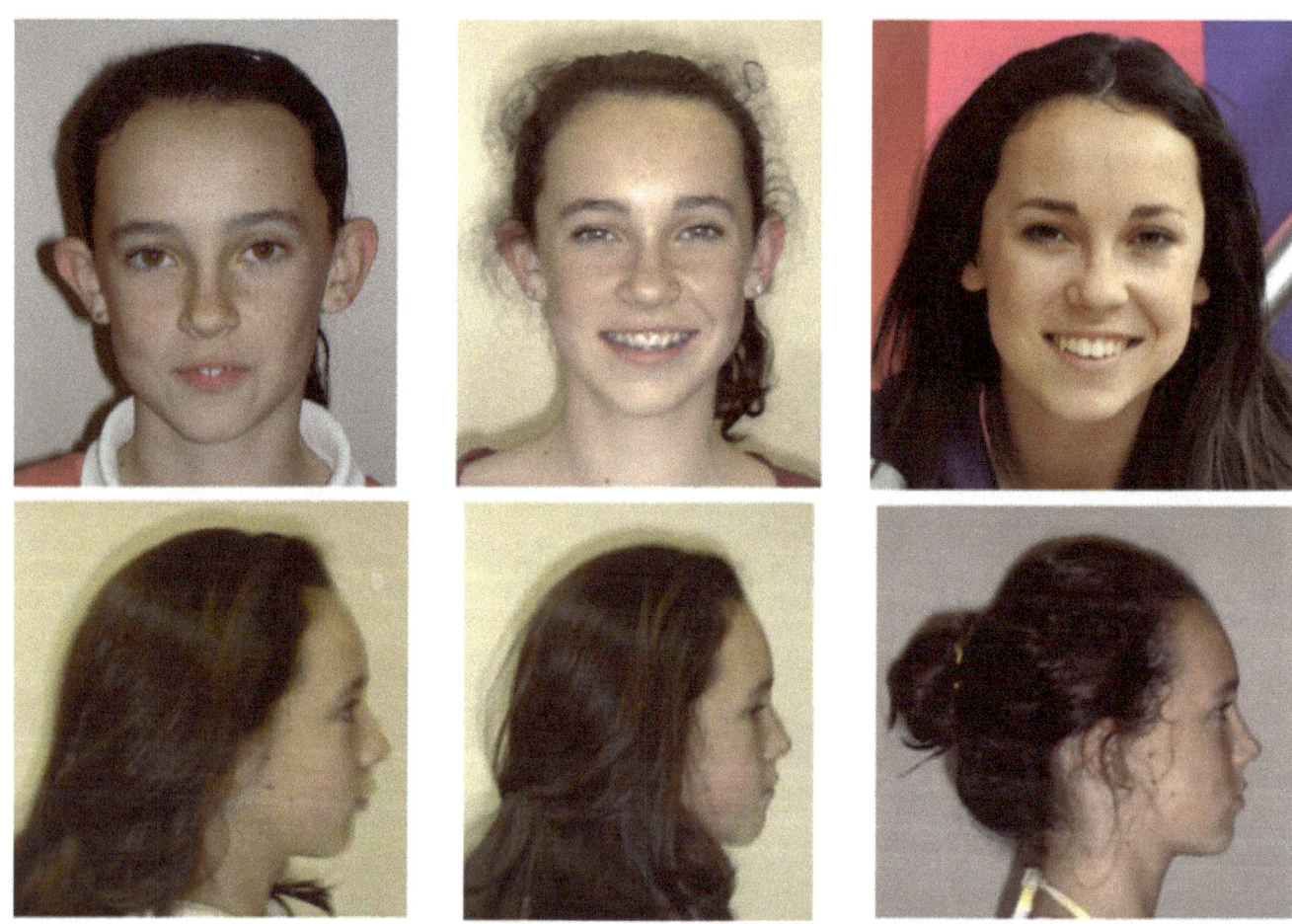

Before treatment   Mandible Postured Forward   After Twin Blocks

FIXED TWIN BLOCKS IN POST PUBERTAL STAGE

This 18 year old girl has a Class II malocclusion and a Class I skeletal relationship with a brachyfacial growth pattern in the post pubertal stage of development. The overjet is 7 mm with a full unit distal occlusion and a narrow upper arch. Secondary crowding in the lower labial segment is due to maxillary contraction. It was decided to correct the distal occlusion as the first step in treatment.

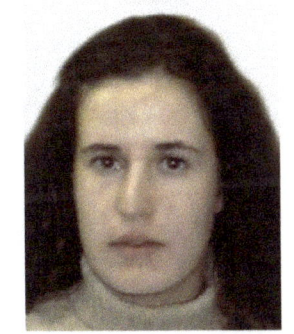
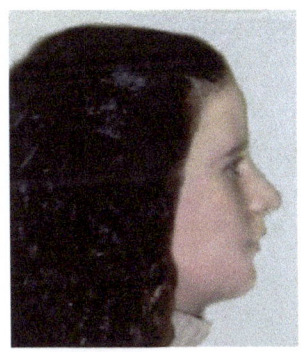

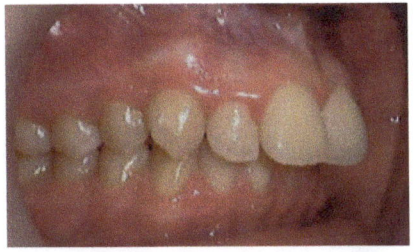
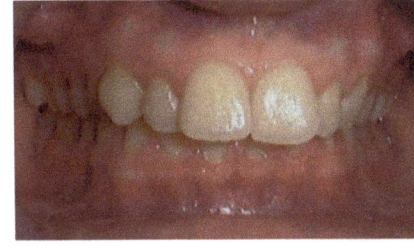
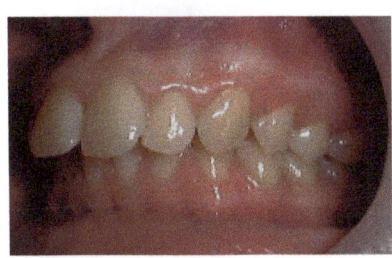

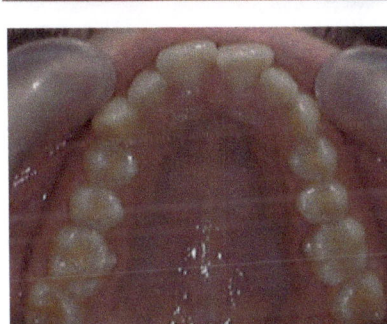
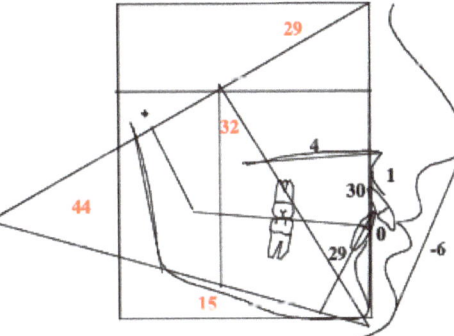
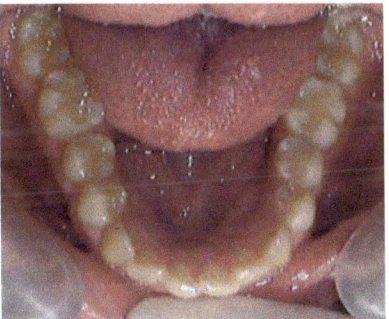

Before Treatment: Cranial Base Angle 29 °: Facial Axis 32 °: Mandibular Plane 15 ° Convexity 1 mm

Fixed Twin Blocks were fitted as the first step in treatment. The profile photos show the profile before treatment. The middle photograph is before treatment with the mandible postured forward with the lips closed. This is a preview of the end result and is similar to the profile on the right when the Fixed Twin Blocks are fitted.

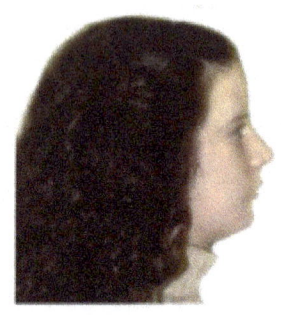 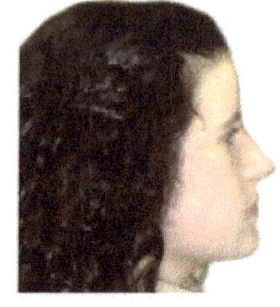 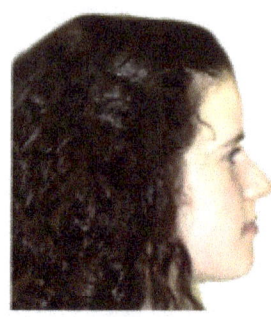

Before treatment   Mandible postured forward   Twin Blocks Fitted

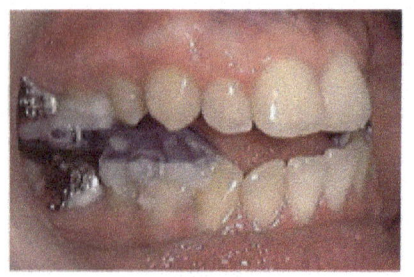 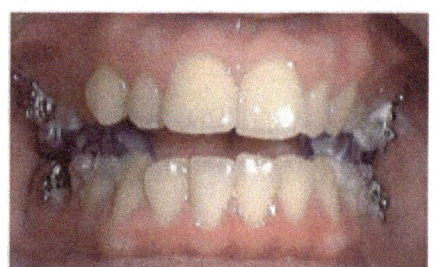 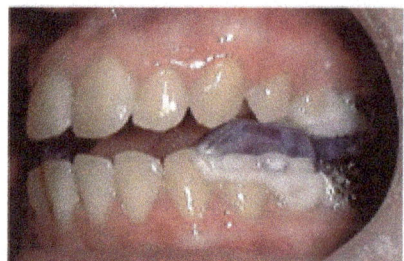

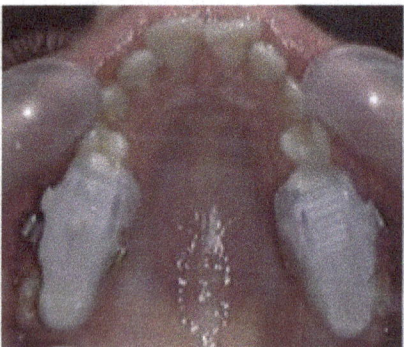 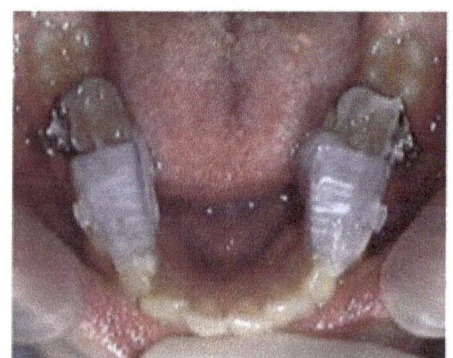

Profile changes are reinforced as we pass through treatment. Fixed Twin Blocks are removed after 8 months treatment. Vertical box elastics are applied to close the slight posterior open bite. At this stage there is little improvement in the alignment of the lower anterior teeth and progress is slow. Arch development is required to relieve anterior crowding.

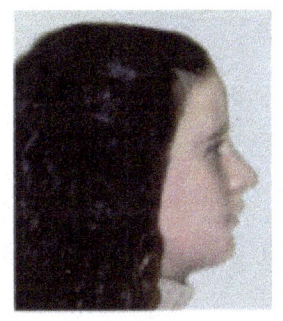 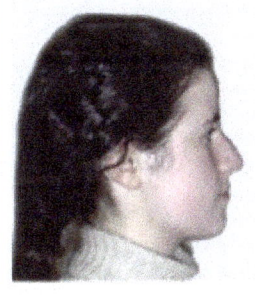 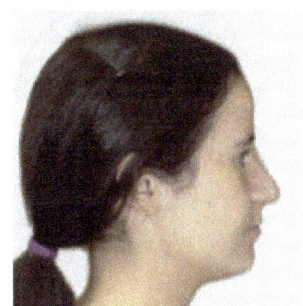

Before treatment   2 Months treatment   8 Months treatment

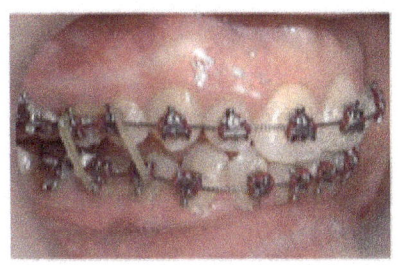 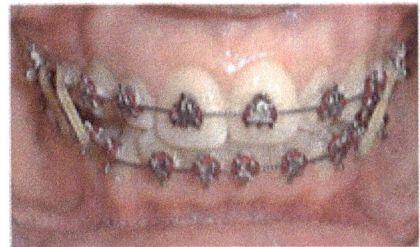 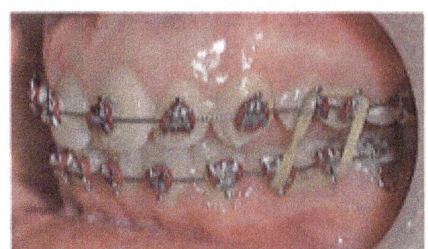

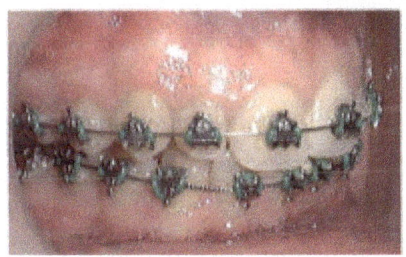 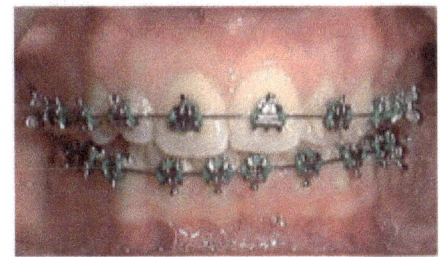 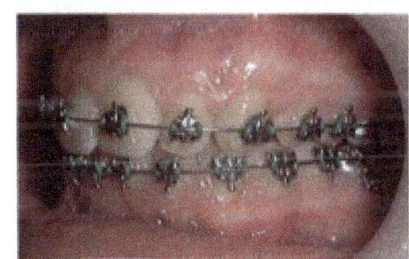

153

Transforce appliances are fitted to expand the arch form and provide space to align the upper and lower anterior teeth. After 14 months treatment fixed/functional therapy has corrected the distal occlusion to a class I relationship and treatment is continuing with fixed appliances to detail the occlusion.

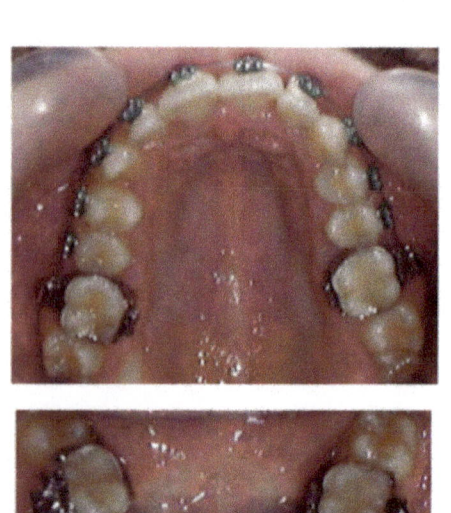
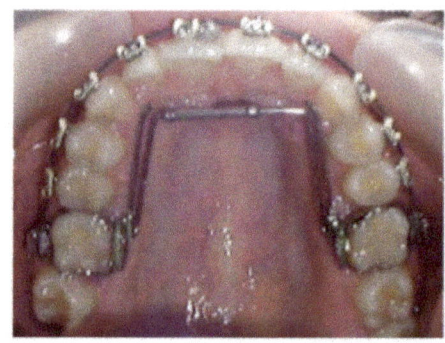
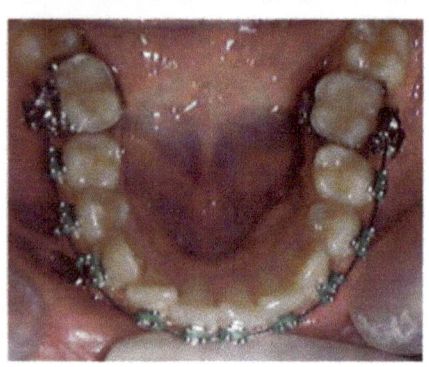
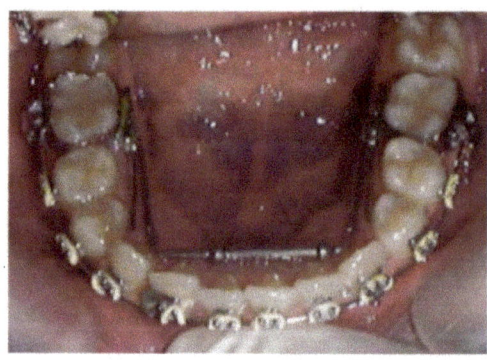
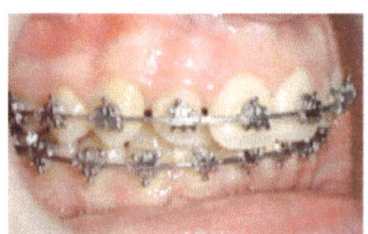
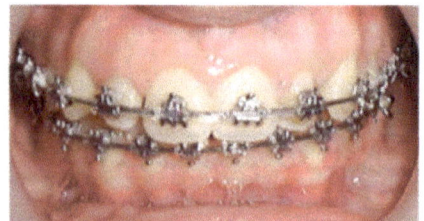
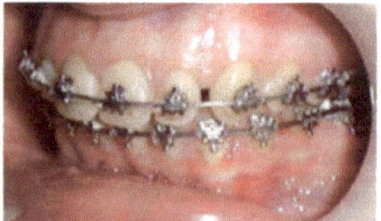

The fixed appliance phase, including arch development extended over a period of 2 years. After removal of the Fixed Twin Blocks treatment continued with Straight Wire Technique, but correction of lower labial crowding was slow until Transforce appliances were fitted to create space to align the teeth. Final records show the position on removal of the fixed appliances before fitting fixed lingual retainers.

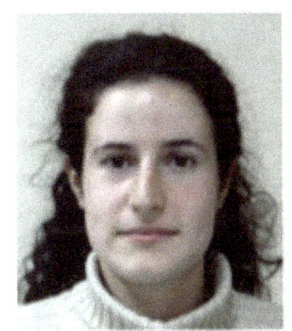
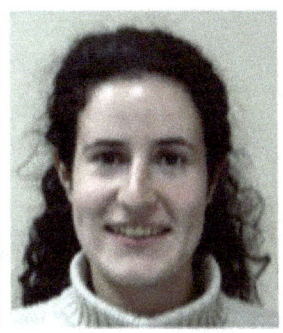
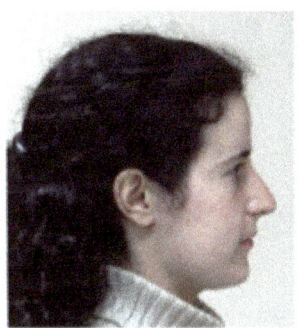

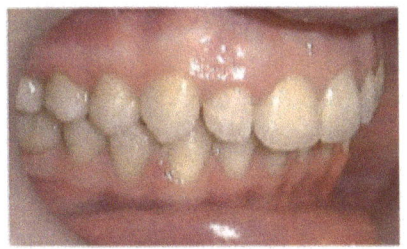
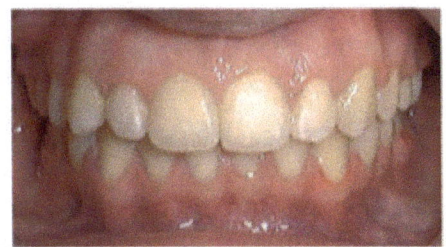
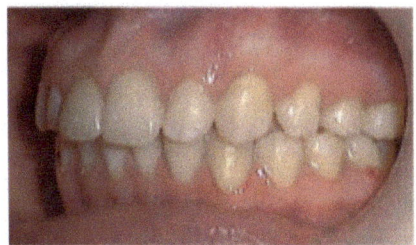

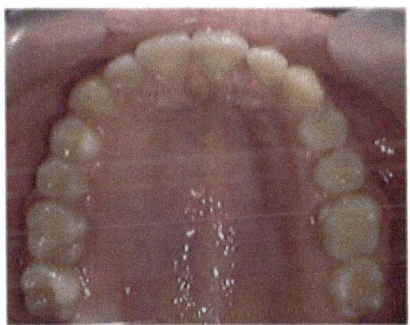
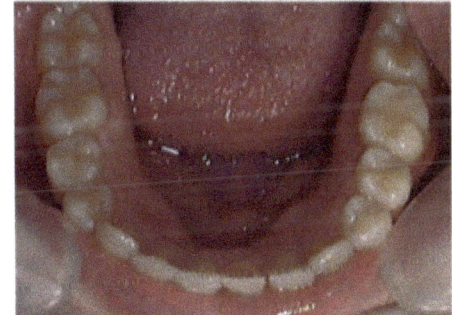

Chapter 9

Carriere ® Self Ligating Brackets

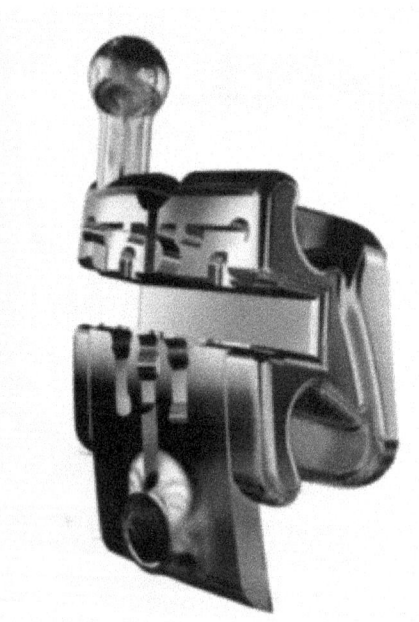 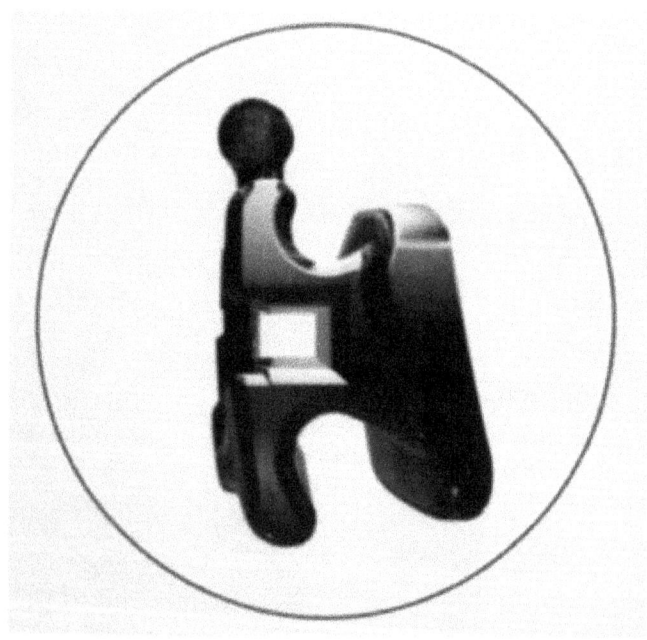

 The Carriere® bracket is an innovative system developed by Dr Luis Carriere in his orthodontic practice in Barcelona. It has a friction fit locking mechanism with a lock that slides open towards the occlusal edge of the tooth. This has the advantage of a low profile that does not accommodate a spring mechanism and is therefore comfortable for the patient. The locking mechanism is simple and effective, using a pointed tool to slide the lock open and it is closed by finger pressure.

COLOR CODED

CARRIERE BRACKET
IDENTIFICATION SYSTEM

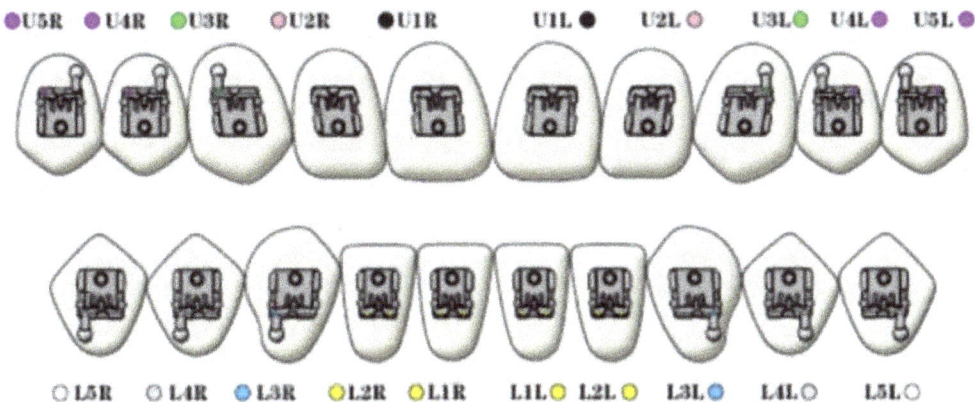

●U5R ●U4R ●U3R ⊙U2R ●U1R   U1L ●   U2L ⊙   U3L● U4L● U5L●

○L5R   ○L4R   ●L3R   ○L2R   ○L1R   L1L○ L2L○   L3L●   L4L○   L5L○

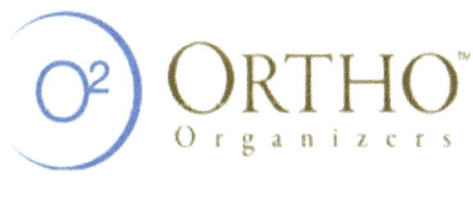

1. Adhesive Application

Use your favorite self cure or light cure adhesive. No change in your current bonding technique is required.

Carriere LX has a micro-etched bonding base for increased bond strength.

2. Positioning

Because of its rhomboid shape, the bracket is easily lined up with the long axis of the clinical crown.

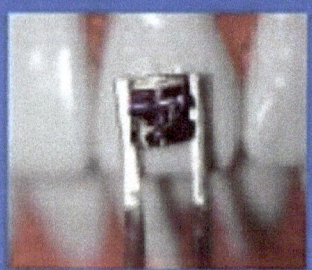

Position bracket on tooth.

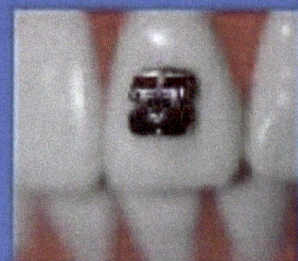

Brackets are individually color-coded for easy identification.

3. Opening Locking Mechanism

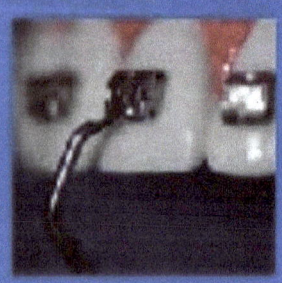 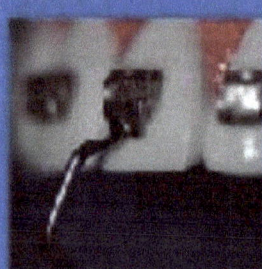

Place tip of Cap Opener Double Wire Director (or instrument such as an explorer) in opening and apply light downward pressure.

4. Seating of The Archwire

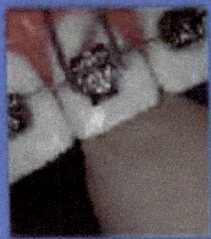
Use the forked end of a double wire director to help seat wire.

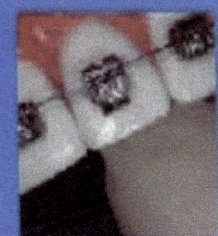
Fully engage wire before closing the locking mechanism.

5. Closing Locking Mechanism

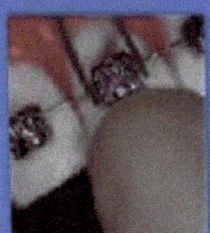
Close the locking mechanism by pressing upward with your finger.

6. Deep Bite Cases

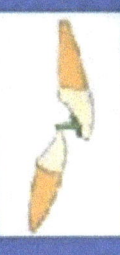
For deep bite cases, a bite guide is recommended prior to placing on lower anteriors.

For additional product information, please visit **www.OrthoOrganizers.com** or call customer service at 800.547.2000 or 760.471.0206.

Opening the bracket

Closing the bracket

Placing the archwire

Open all the bracket slots before applying the archwire

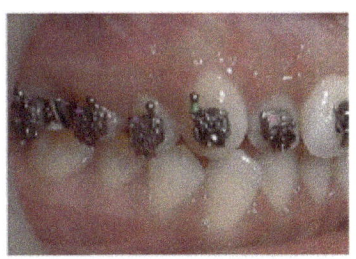
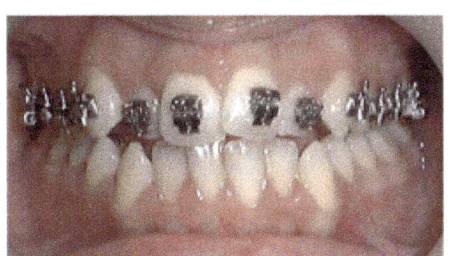
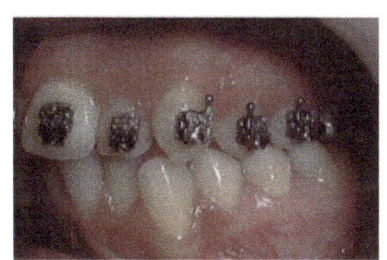

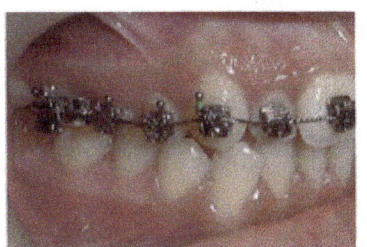
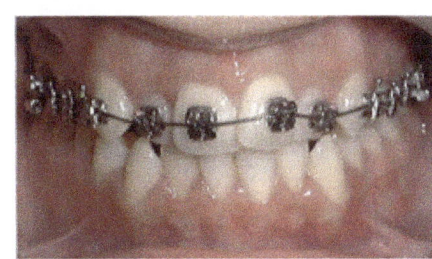
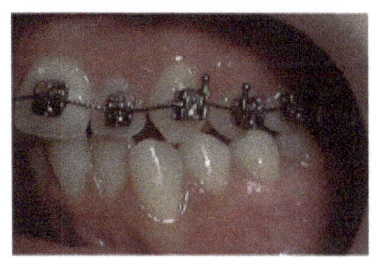

Brackets can be combined with TransForce lingual appliances for arch development

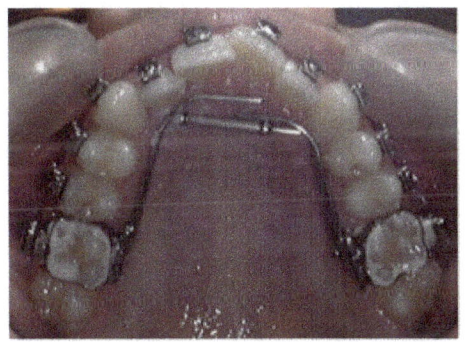
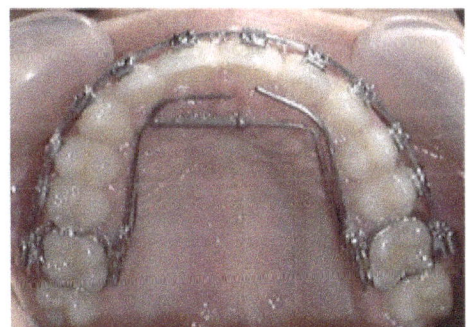

ADULT THERAPY

CARRIERE® SELF LIGATING BRACKETS

A 26 Year old adult attended with chronic TMJ pain and dysfunction relating to a Class I occlusion. with premature contacts on third molars, which were removed before treatment. She had a severe click and mandibular displacement to the left on opening and closing, indicating that the disc was consistently displaced off the condyle and recaptured late in the opening movement.

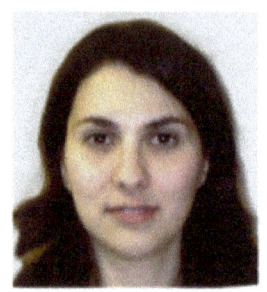 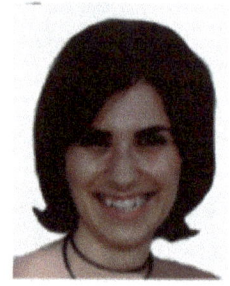 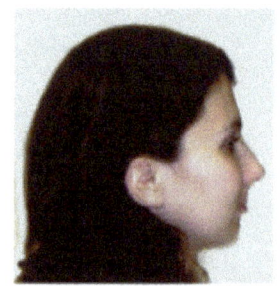

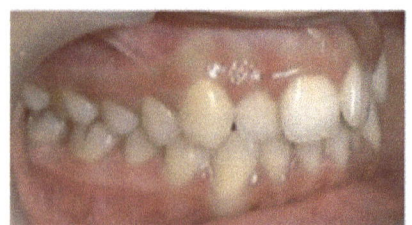 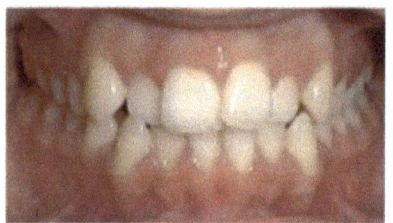 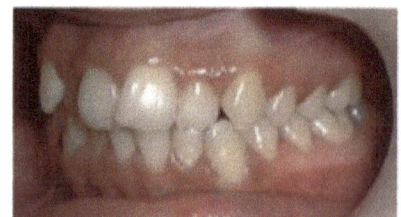

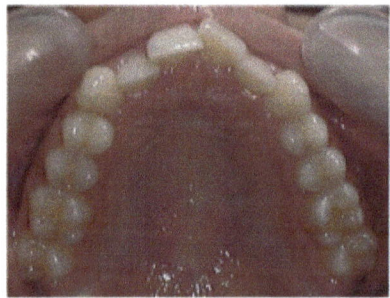 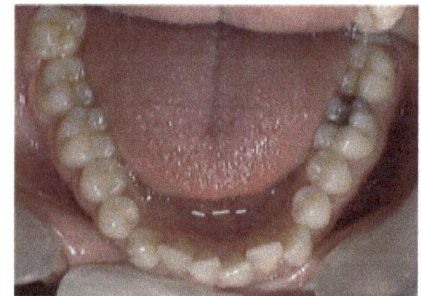

An upper TransForce lingual appliance was fitted for transverse expansion. Expanding the upper inter-canine width helped to relieve pressure on the lower labial segment. This combination of light forces from the lingual aspect for arch development works very well to create space and control anterior crowding in synergy with a fixed appliance to detail the occlusion. The TransForce appliance remained in place throughout treatment to act as a retainer after transverse expansion.

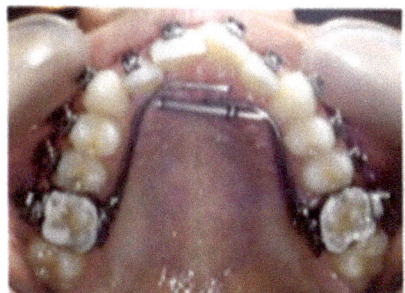
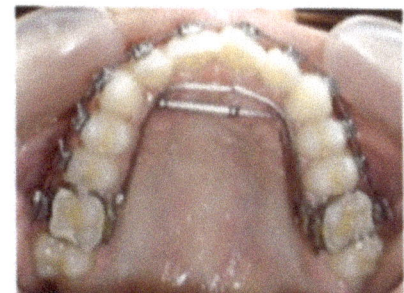
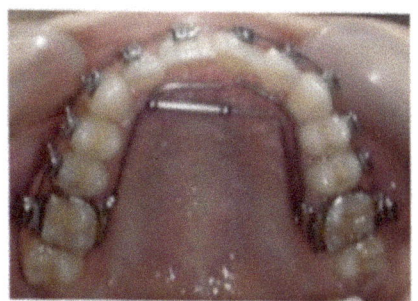

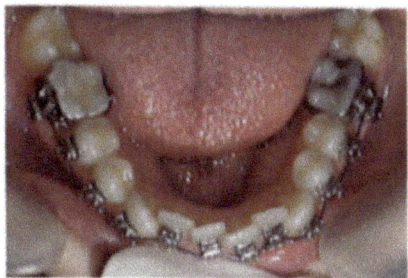
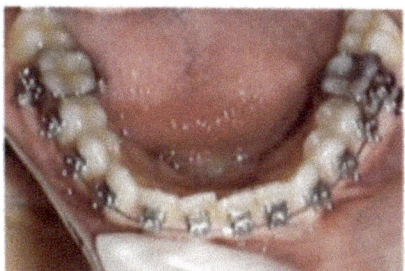
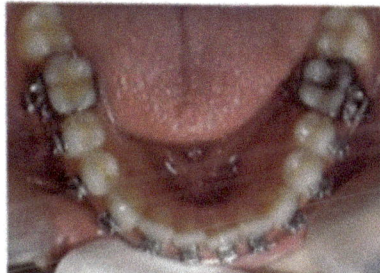

An upper TransForce lingual appliance was fitted for transverse expansion. Expanding the upper inter-canine width helped to relieve pressure on the lower labial segment. This combination of light forces from the lingual aspect for arch development works very well to create space and control anterior crowding in synergy with a fixed appliance to detail the occlusion. The TransForce appliance remained in place throughout treatment to act as a retainer after transverse expansion.

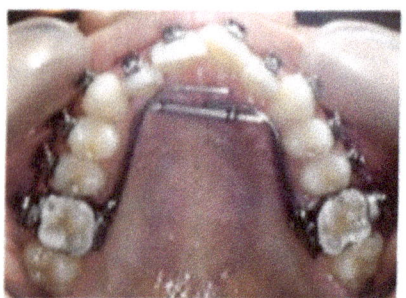
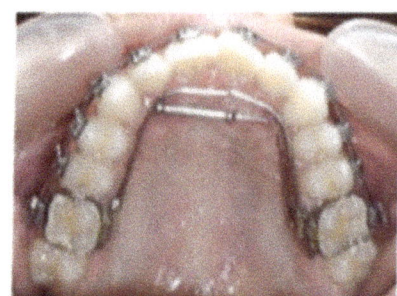
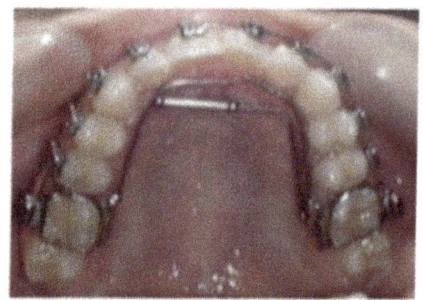
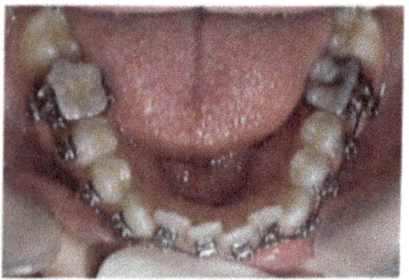
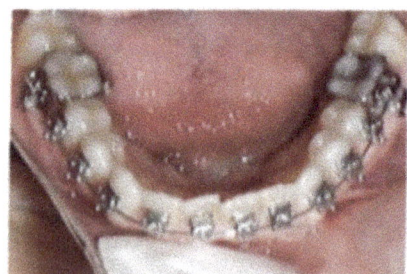
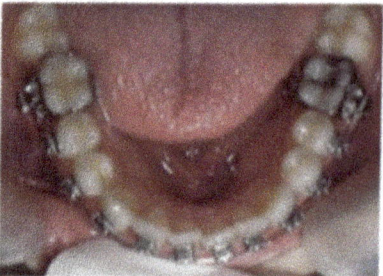

Articulating paper was used to check for premature contacts on the posterior teeth and selective grinding of the first and second molars helped to balance the occlusion. Active treatment was completed in two years and ten appointments.

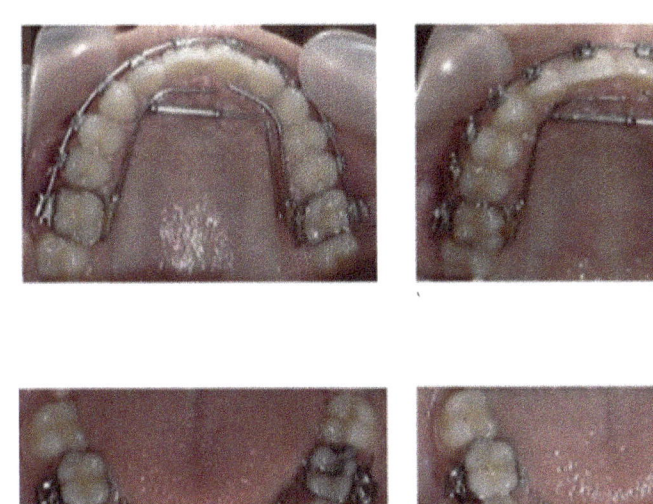
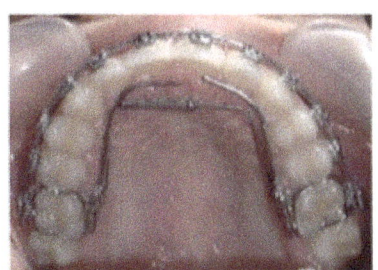
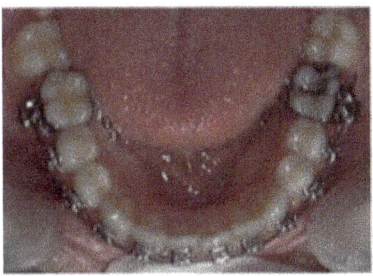
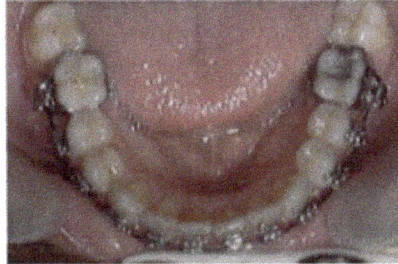
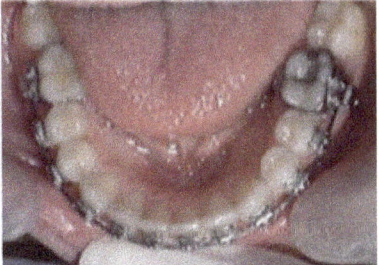

Before treatment there appears to be little bony support labial to the lower incisors and this, together with the temporomandibular joint pain and displacement this requires careful management. It is important to apply light forces and take adequate time between changing arch wires. Carriere SLB (self ligating brackets) were used to deliver light controlled forces to achieve a balanced functional occlusion. This series shows the sequence of arch wire changes. Appointments were at 10 week intervals.

Fitted Upper Appliance: .018 Supercable

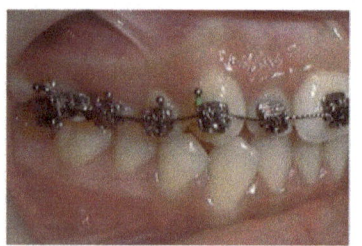 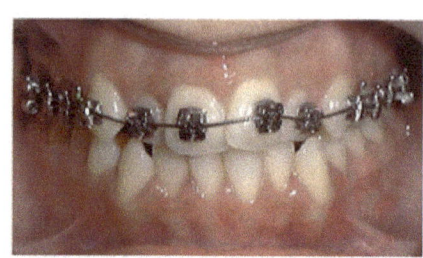 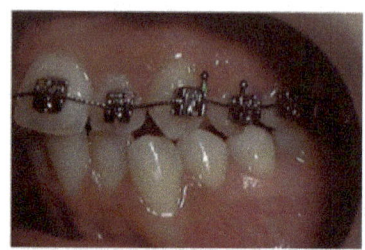

2 Months Treatment - Fitted Lower Appliance: .018 Supercable

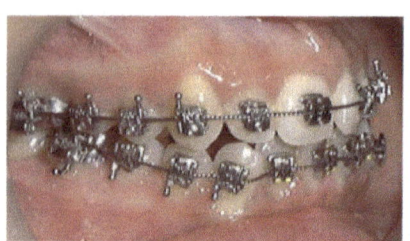 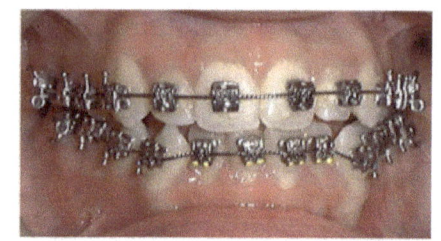 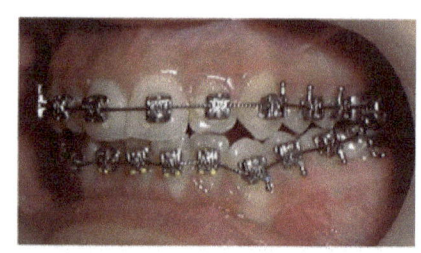

5 Months Treatment U .016 X .022: L ,016 X .016 Nitinol

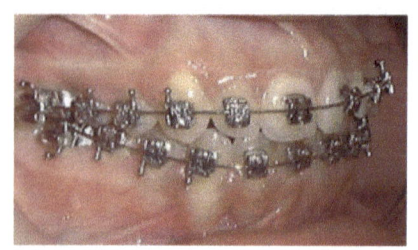 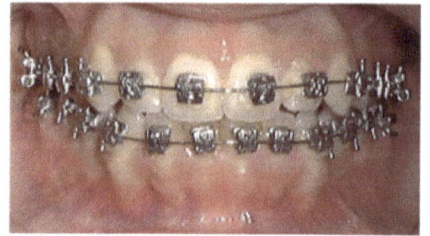 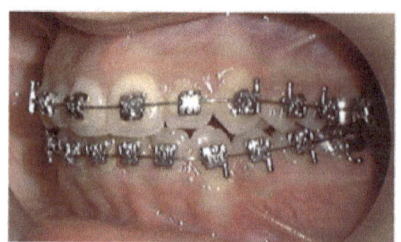

Resolving the patient's chronic pain was the main objective of treatment. The Temporo mandibular joint pain eased during treatment and the loud click on displacement of the disc was resolved. It is also necessary to check tooth mobility and periodontal condition throughout the treatment. There were no undue problems with tooth mobility and the patient maintained good oral hygiene to help the periodontal condition.

10 Months Treatment U/L .016 X .022 Nitinol

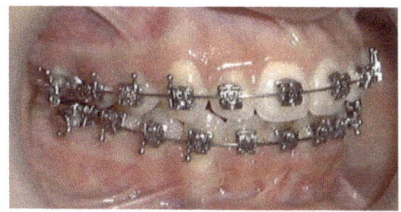 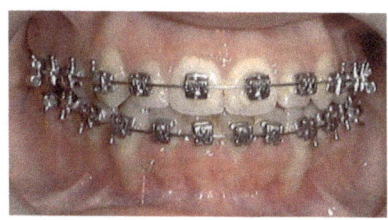 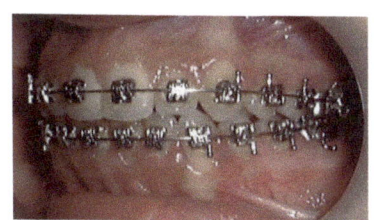

12 Months Treatment U/L .017 X .025 Nitinol

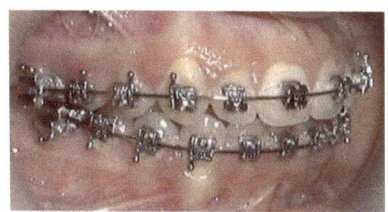 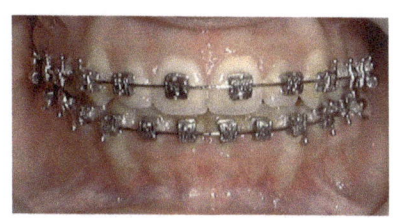 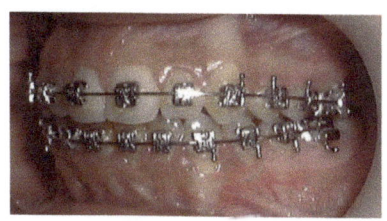

18 Months Treatment U/L .019 X .025 Stainless Steel

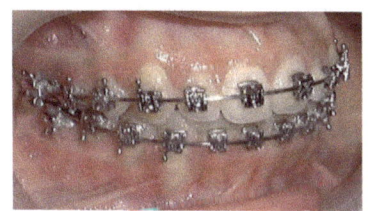 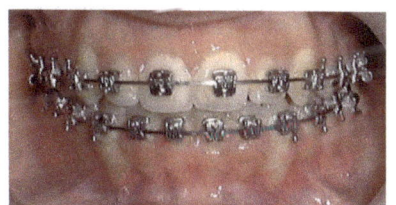 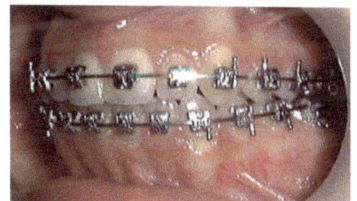

Cranial Base Angle 29°: Facial Axis 21°: Mandibular Plane 39° Convexity 6 mm

The chronic mandibular joint pain and mandibular displacement appeared to be related to premature contact on the lower right third molar and all third molars were removed before treatment. A high mandibular plane angle of 39° presented a challenging dolichofacial pattern. The patient responded well to treatment and removal of the third molars appeared to help in relieving the joint symptoms and balancing the occlusion.

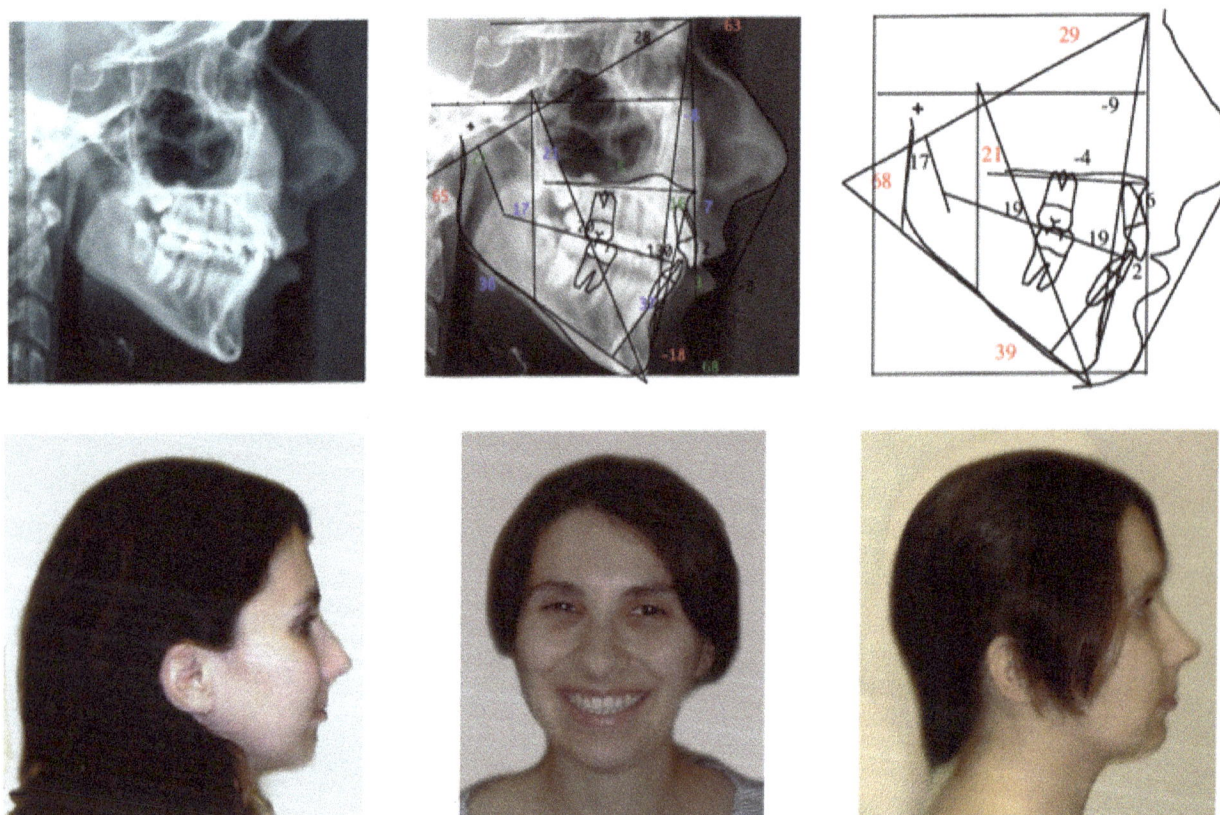

The patient is now pain free and the click has virtually disappeared. Removable retainers were fitted first with fixed retainers to follow. The gingival condition has improved and there is no mobility of the teeth.

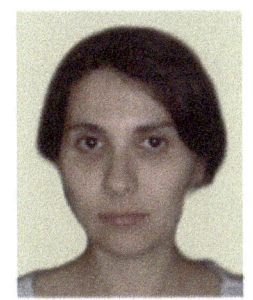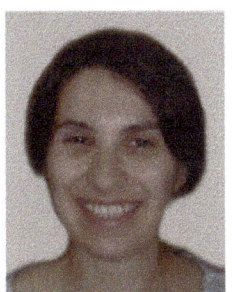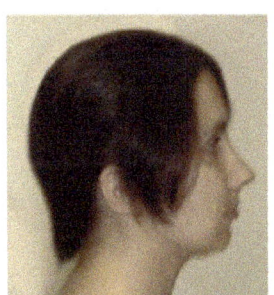

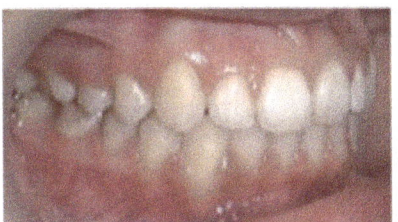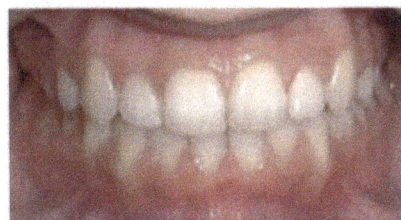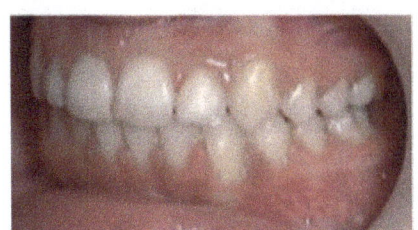

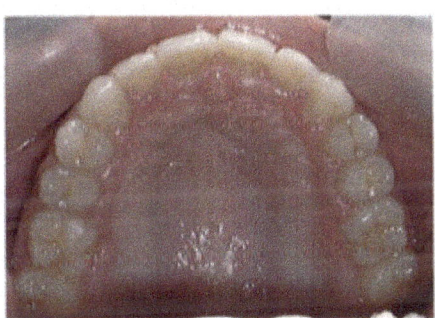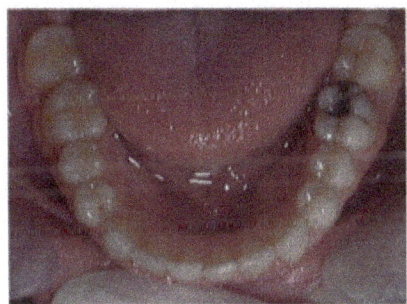

169

In Retention after 2 Years' Treatment - 10 Appointments

Improved technology continues to advance the sophistication of contemporary orthodontic technique. Aesthetic brackets are especially important in adult therapy. This is an example of adult therapy using NEOLUCENT ceramic brackets that are translucent, and take up the colour of the teeth. This represents the gold standard of aesthetic treatment for adult therapy.

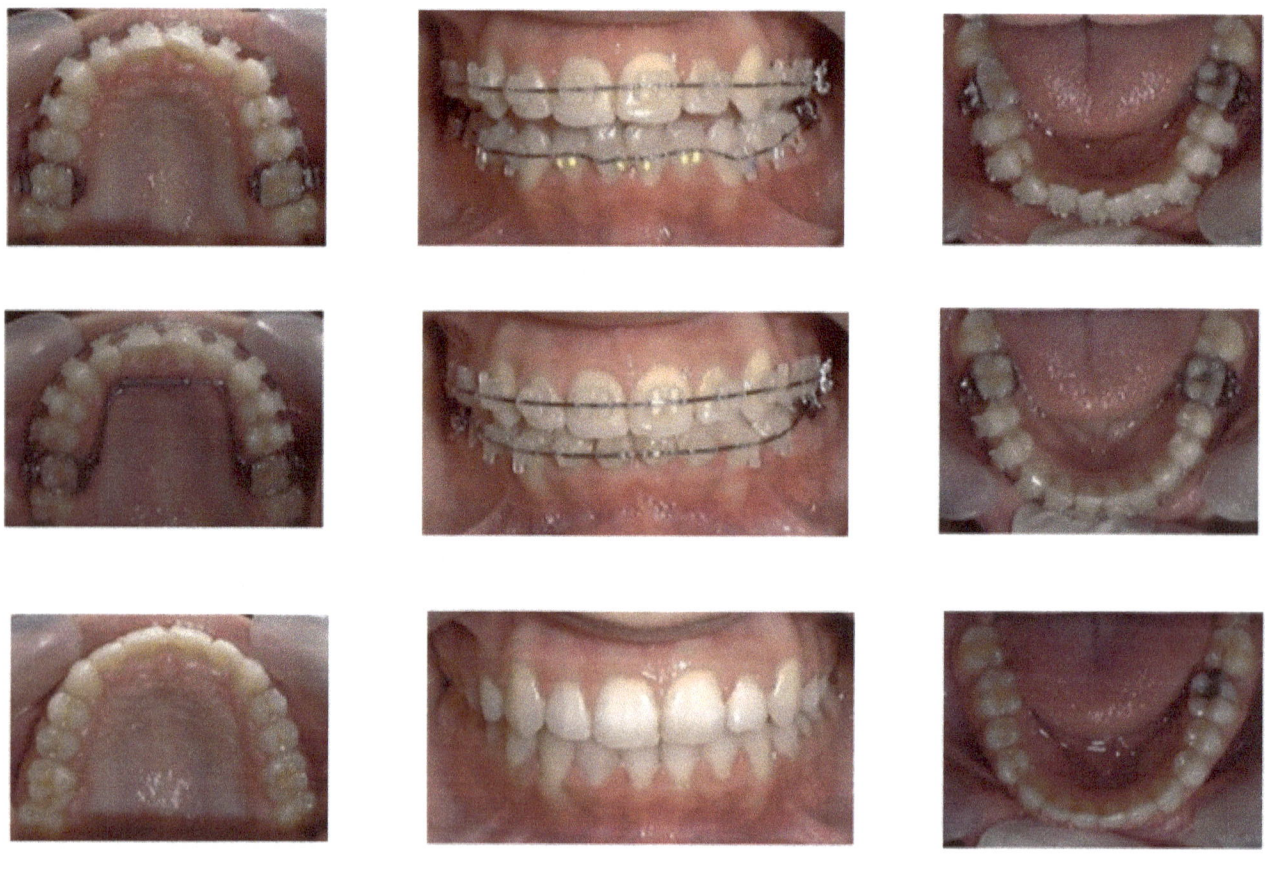

TransForce Combined With Fixed Appliances

This boy presents a Class I malocclusion with narrowing of the upper arch and labial displacement and irregularity of the upper incisors. Upper arch width is reduced and treatment should aim to expand the upper arch to accommodate the permanent canines when they erupt and provide space to align the upper anterior teeth. There is also mild crowding in the lower arch which can be controlled with a lower lingual appliance to maintain space as the remaining permanent teeth erupt.

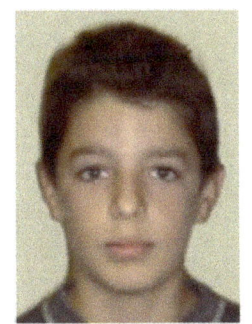
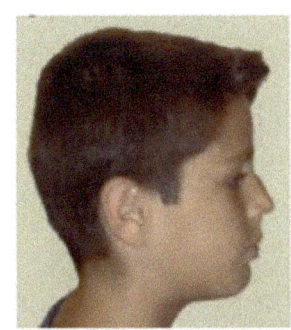

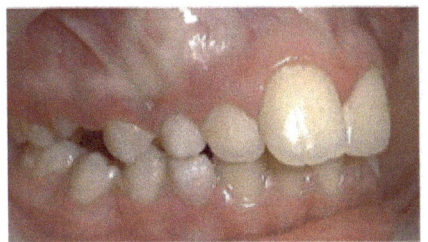
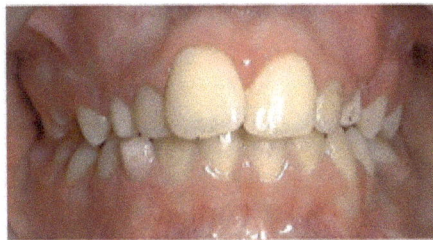
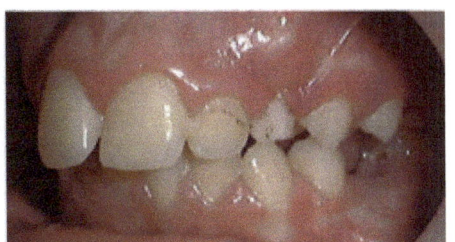

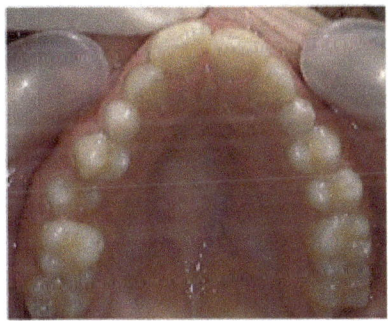
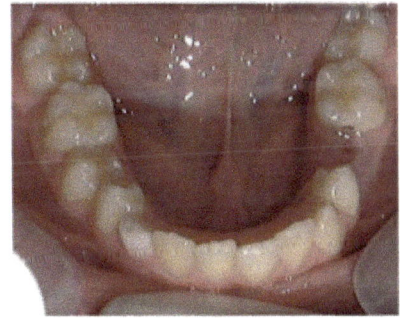

Maxillary expansion with a Transforce appliance effectively changes the vault of the palate from V- shaped to a wider contour. Palatal X-rays show evidence of activity in the mid palatal suture coincident with slow expansion using gentle continuous forces. This concept merits further investigation.

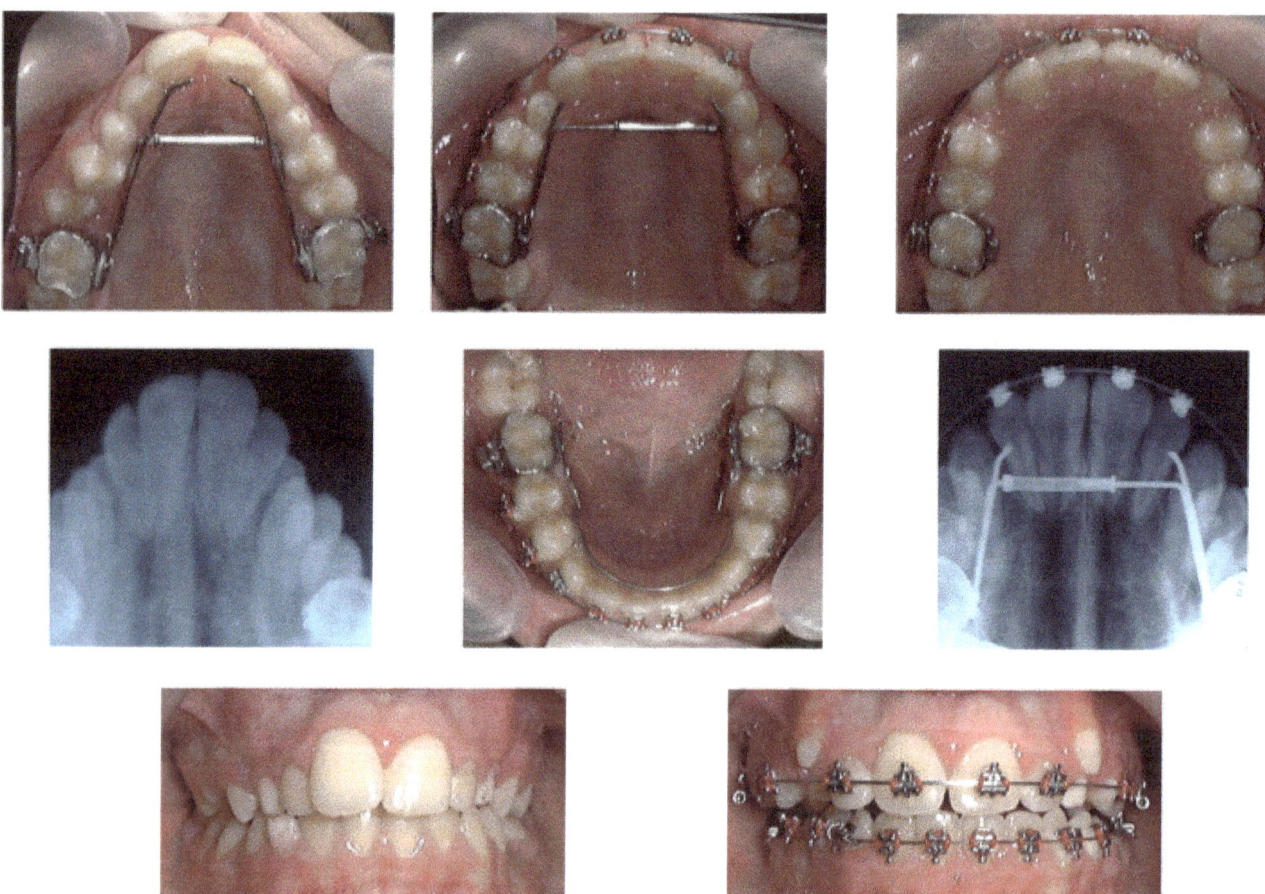

The occlusion has settled at the next visit into a Class I buccal segment relationship. Treatment continues with fixed appliances to detail the occlusion.

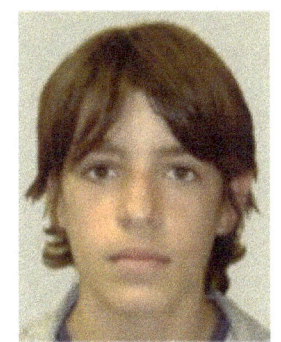 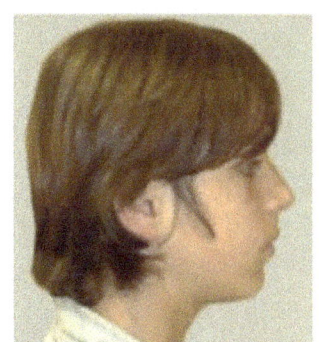

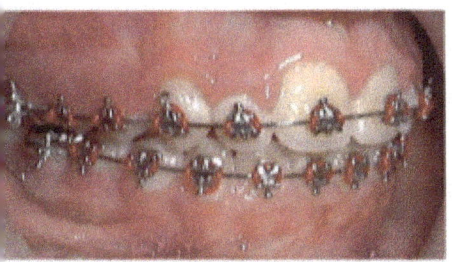 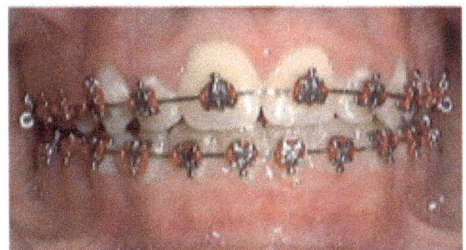 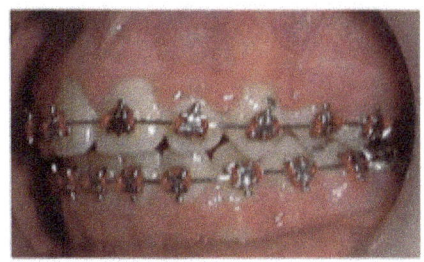

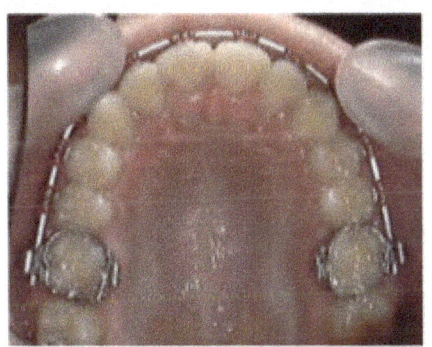 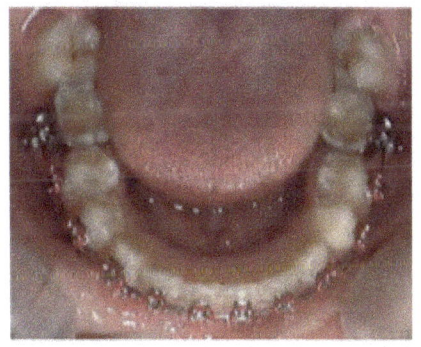

This is followed by an occlusoguide for night time retention. The occlusoguide acts as a functional retainer by posturing the mandible forward to an edge to edge incisor relationship.

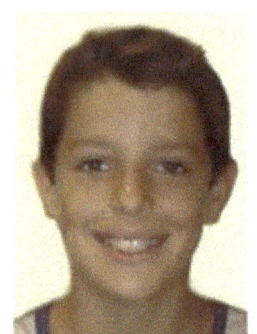 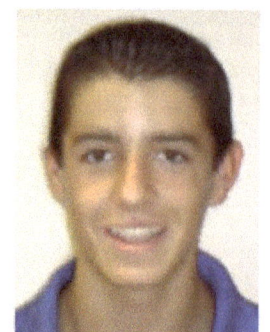

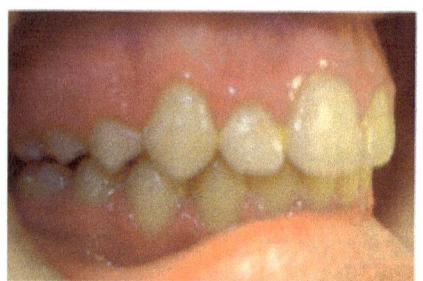 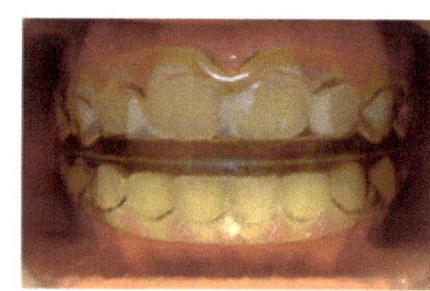 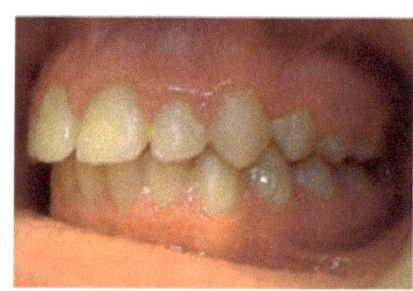

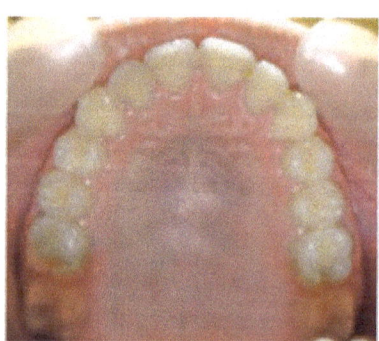 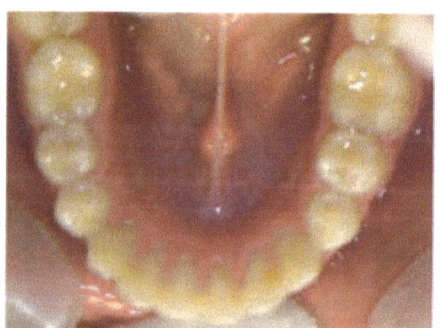

Final records show a slight relapse of the upper incisor irregularity, perhaps because the retention was inadequate. This is referred to as ghosting when the original irregularity returns to a lesser degree than the original condition. this was relatively common,especially in the lower arch before fixed retention was introduced. There are pro's and con's for fixed retainers and the long term effects have still to be confirmed, especially with regard to oral hygiene and periodontal condition.

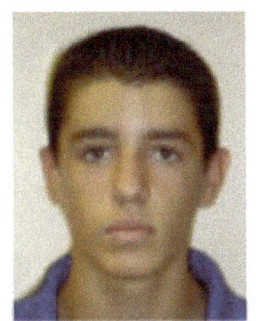
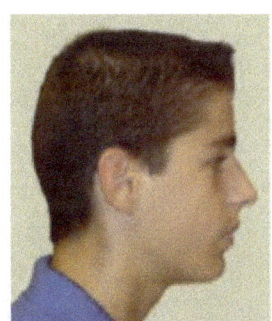

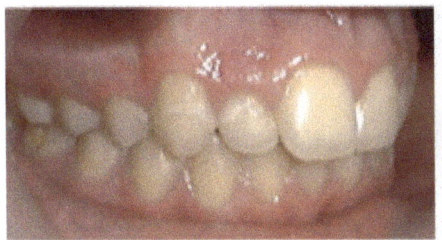
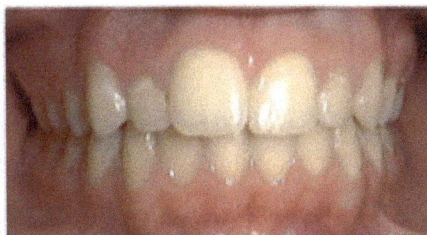
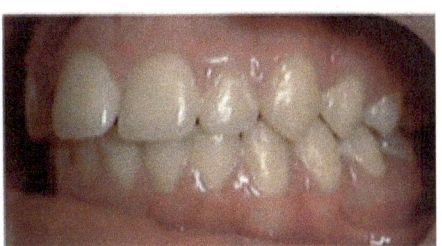

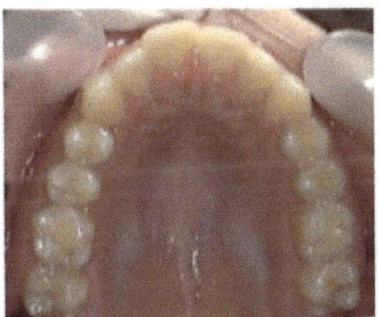
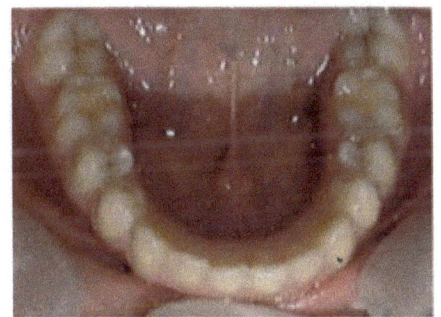

REMOVABLE RETAINERS

Removable retainers were the norm in the latter half of the 20th century. A variety of designs included the Hawley retainer with clasps and labial bows on the anterior teeth, or alternatively a wrap round labial bow extending from the distal of the molars round the arch. The spring retainer uses an acrylic pad to align the incisors, which are first reset on the models. After fixed appliance therapy positioners are customized in the laboratory by cutting the teeth off the model and resetting them for minor adjustment and precise finishing with flexible material.

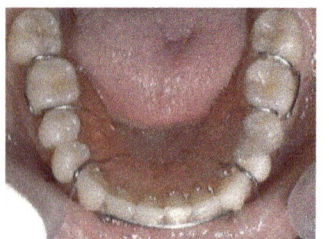 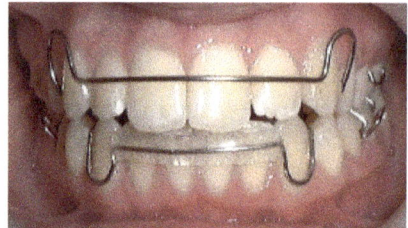 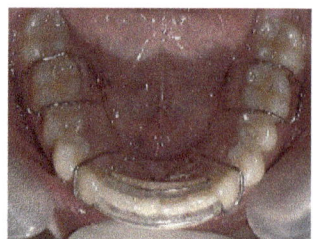

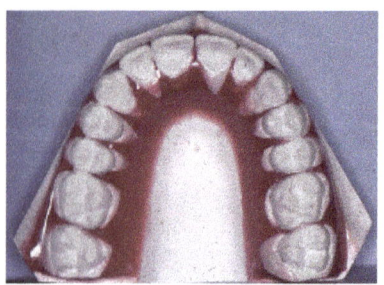 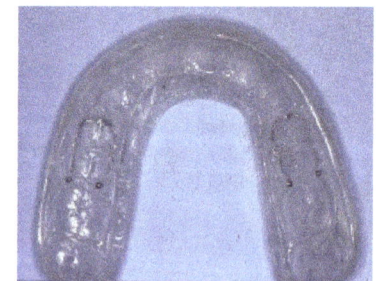 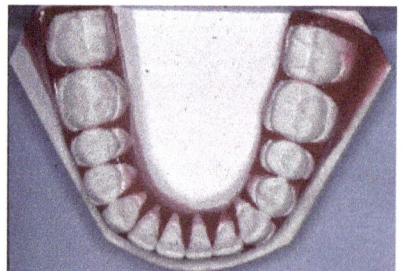

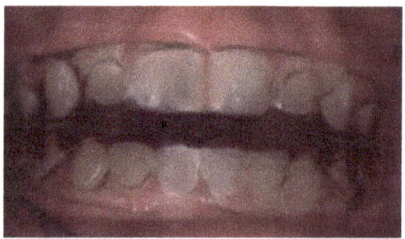 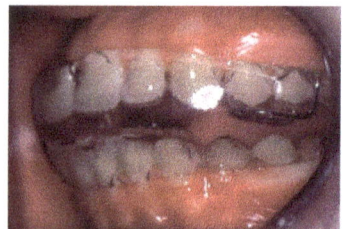

FIXED & INVISIBLE RETAINERS

Frequent recurrence of lower labial crowding resulted in the development of a variety of fixed lingual retainers and invisible retainers for three dimensional control of the anterior teeth after treatment. The objective was to maintain the stability of the corrected occlusion and resist disruptive forces generated by eruption of third molars, or from maturation of labial musculature.

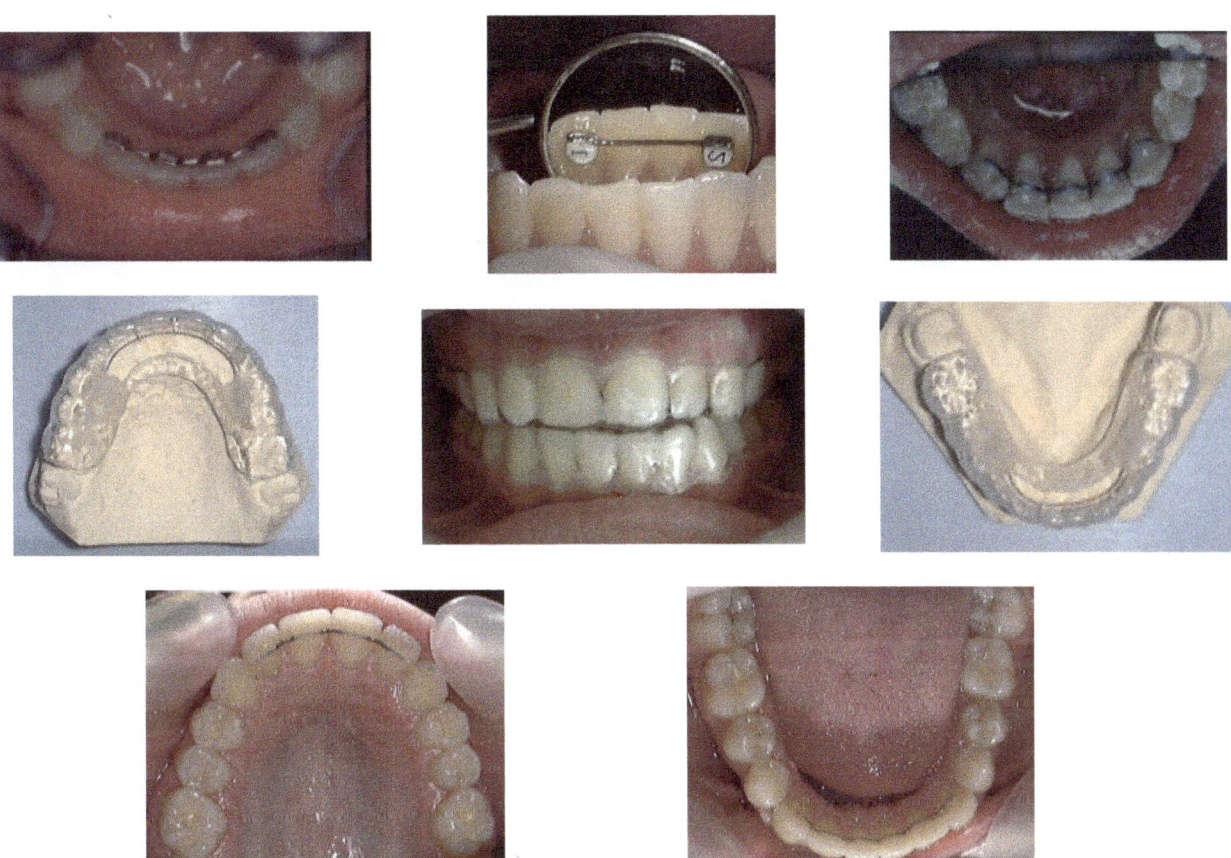

TREATMENT OF LATE CROWDING

A lip bumper was sometimes used to relieve pressure on the lower labial segment from an active mentalis muscle. A lower removable appliance with a midline screw to expand the arch slightly could be used to resolve mild labial crowding, using a labial elastic extended across ball clasps to align the incisors. This can be followed by a fixed lingual retainer

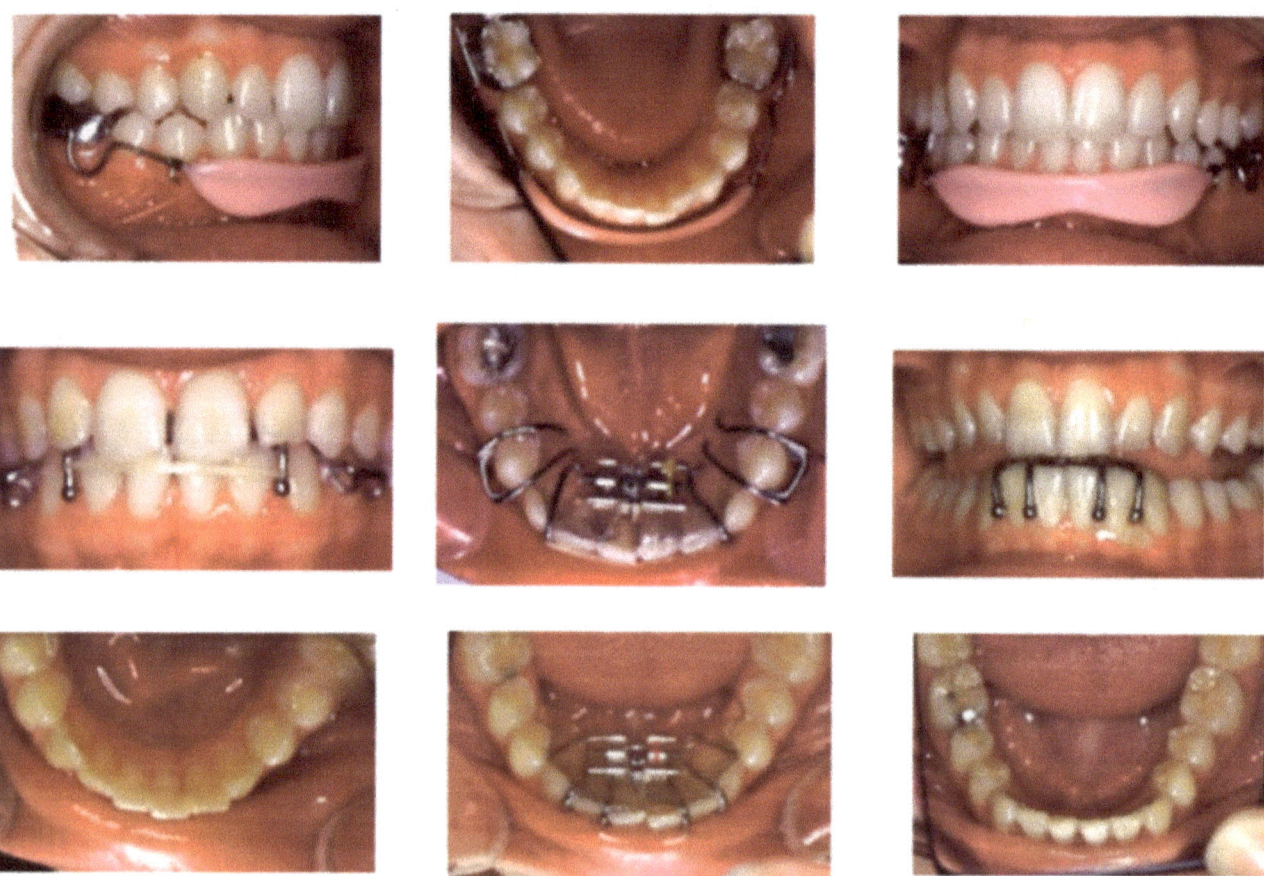

INTERDENTAL STRIPPING

Maintaining the lower inter-canine width is important for stability of the lower labial segment. Minor crowding can be resolved by judicious inter-dental stripping to reduce the combined width of the anterior teeth. Reducing each tooth by 1/4 mm from the mesial of the first premolar is equivalent to 3 mm of crowding. This should be done progressively in the finishing stage of treatment and the final adjustment must be made after the teeth are correctly aligned.

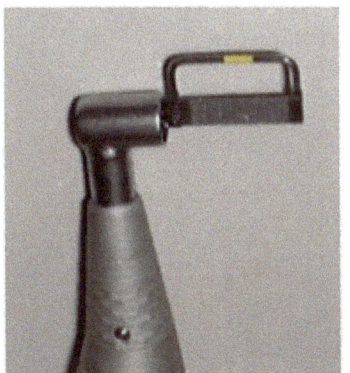
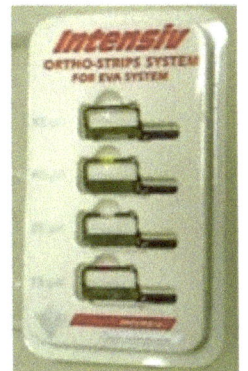
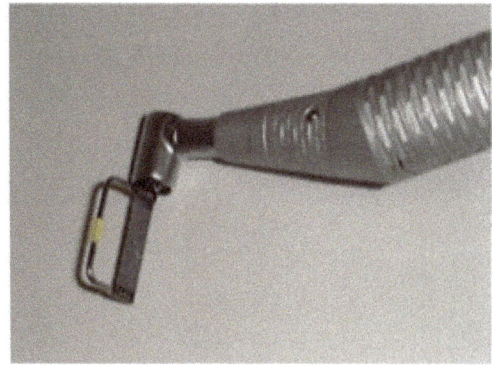

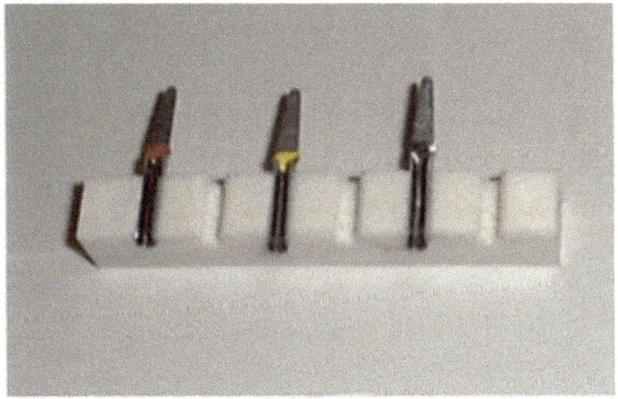
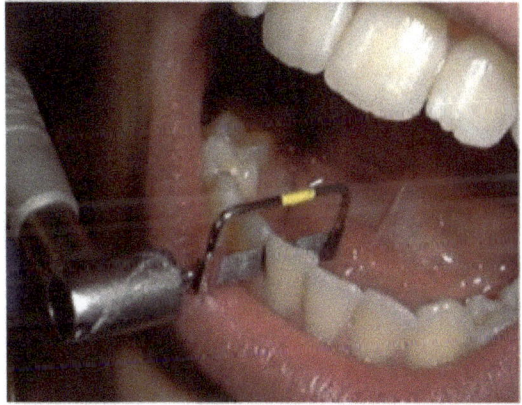

Treatment Of Displaced Canines

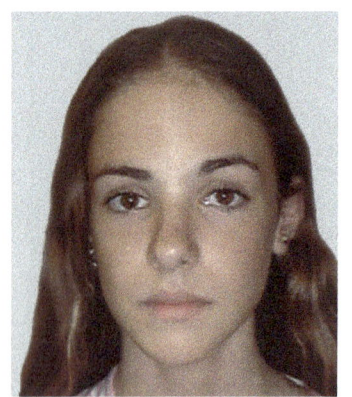
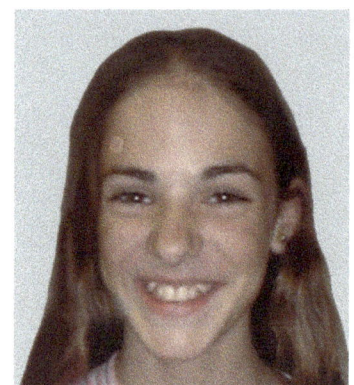
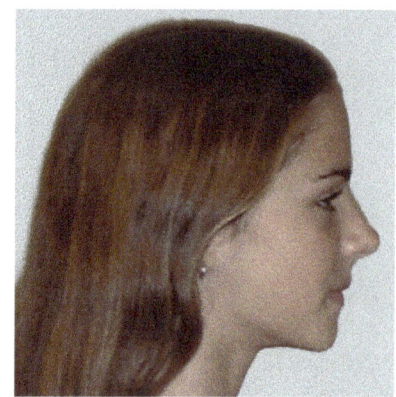

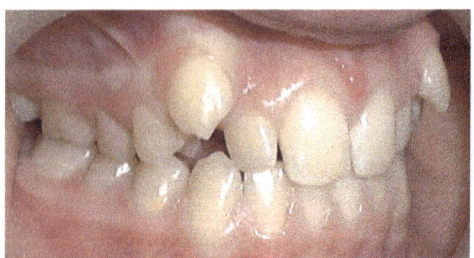
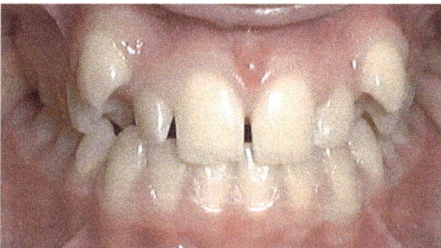
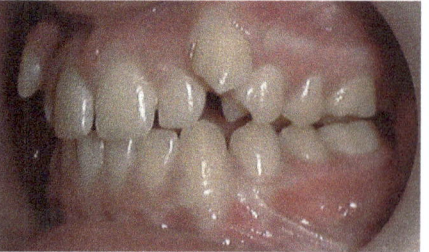

4 Months Treatment - 2 Appointments

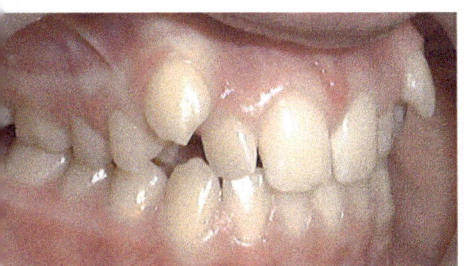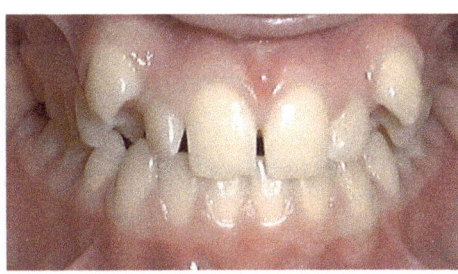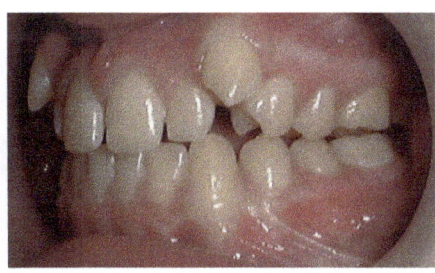

TransForce Palatal Expander

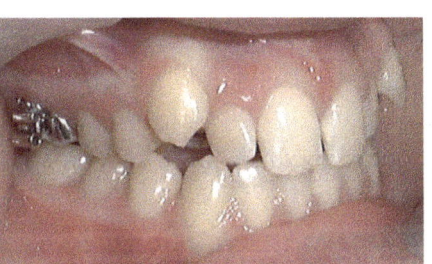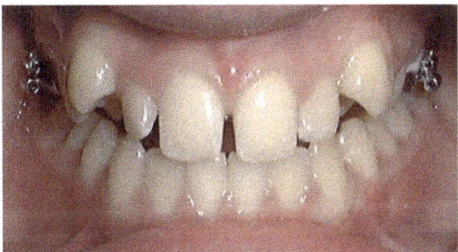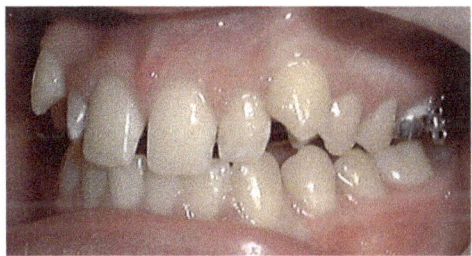

TransForce Orthodontics - 8 Months Treatment

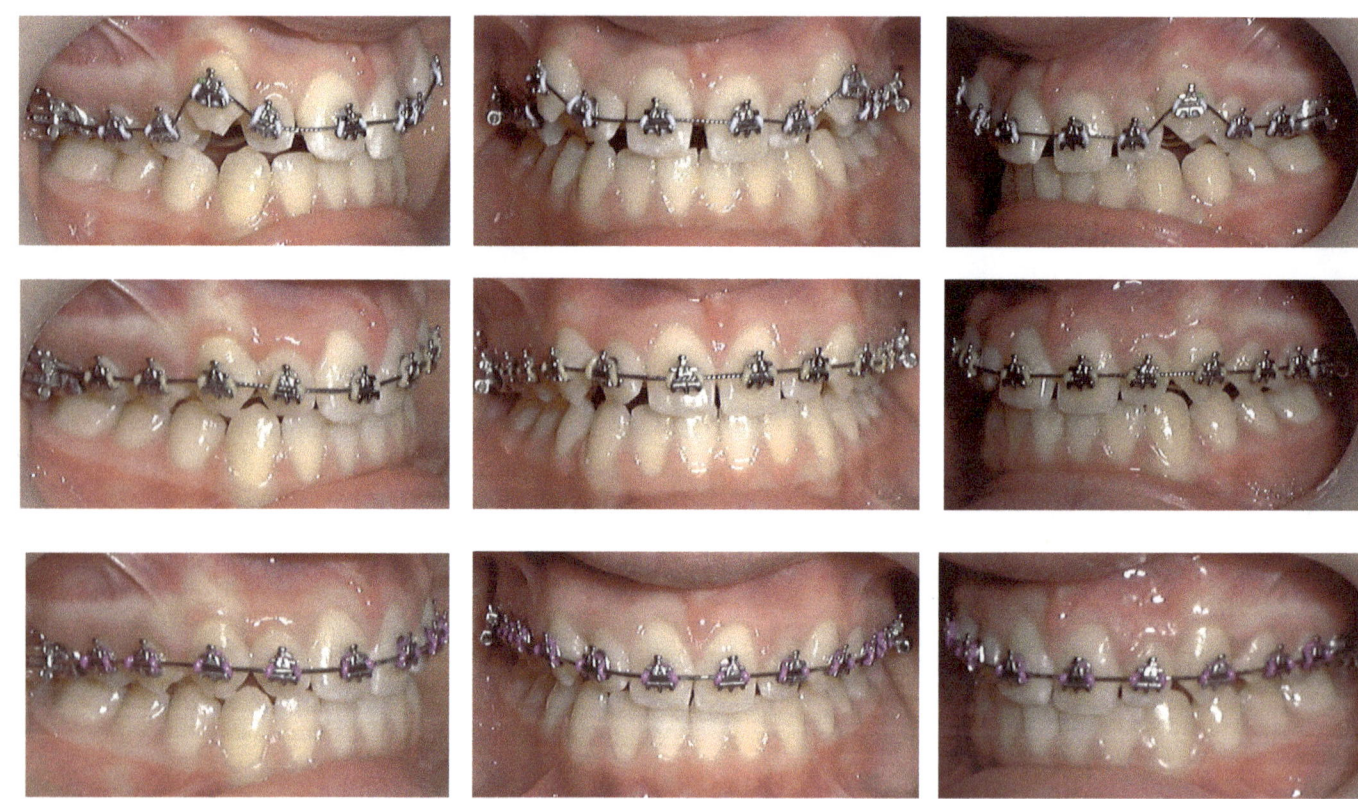

10 Months Treatment - 5 Appointments

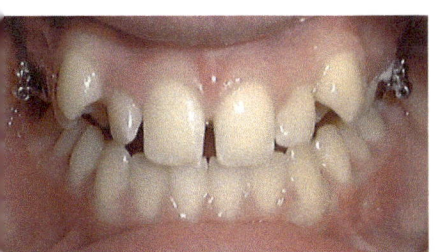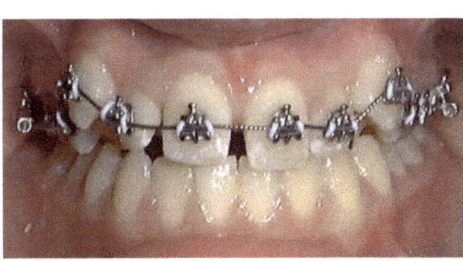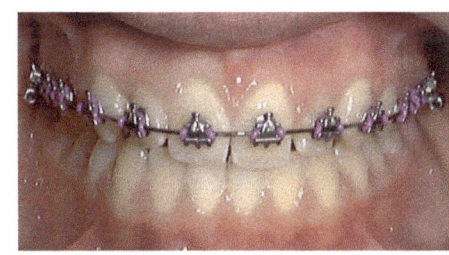

TransForce Palatal Expander with Delta Force Fixed Appliance

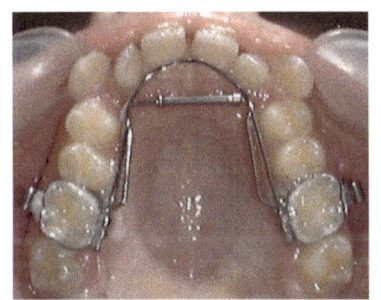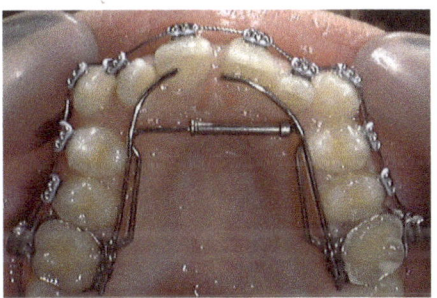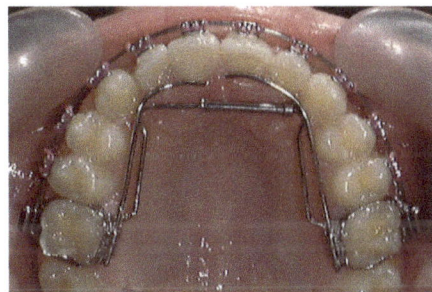

TransForce Palatal Expander Resolves Anterior Crowding

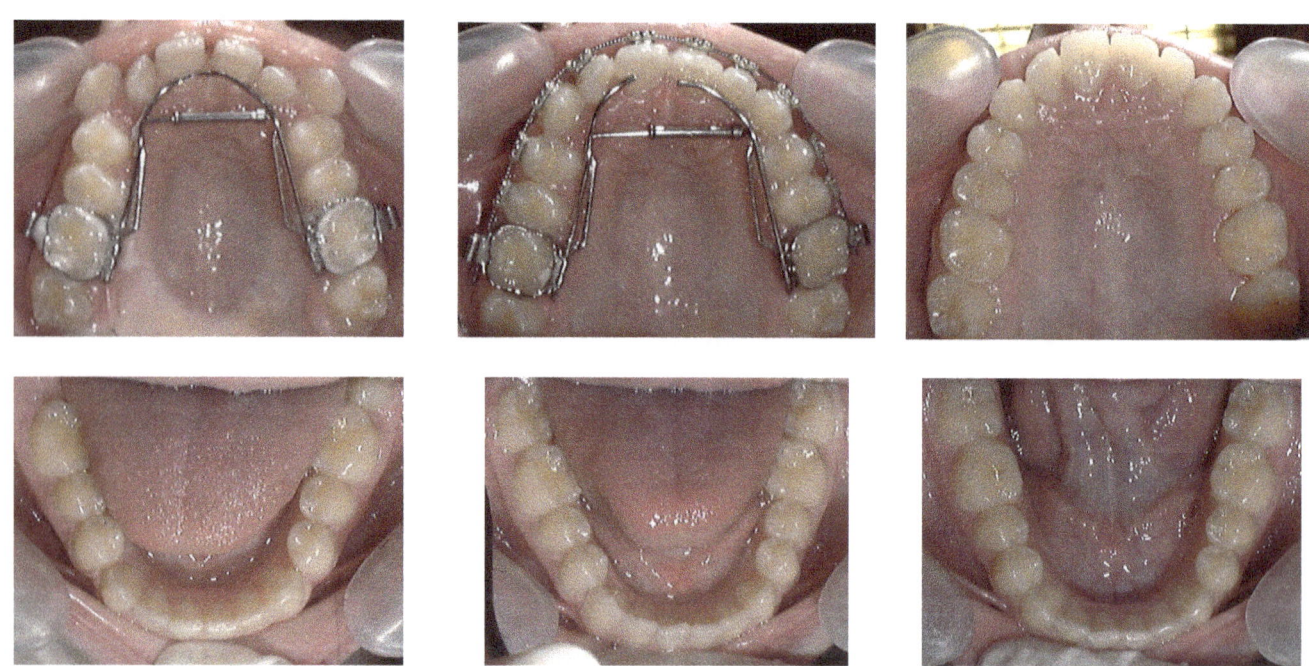

No Lower Appliance Required

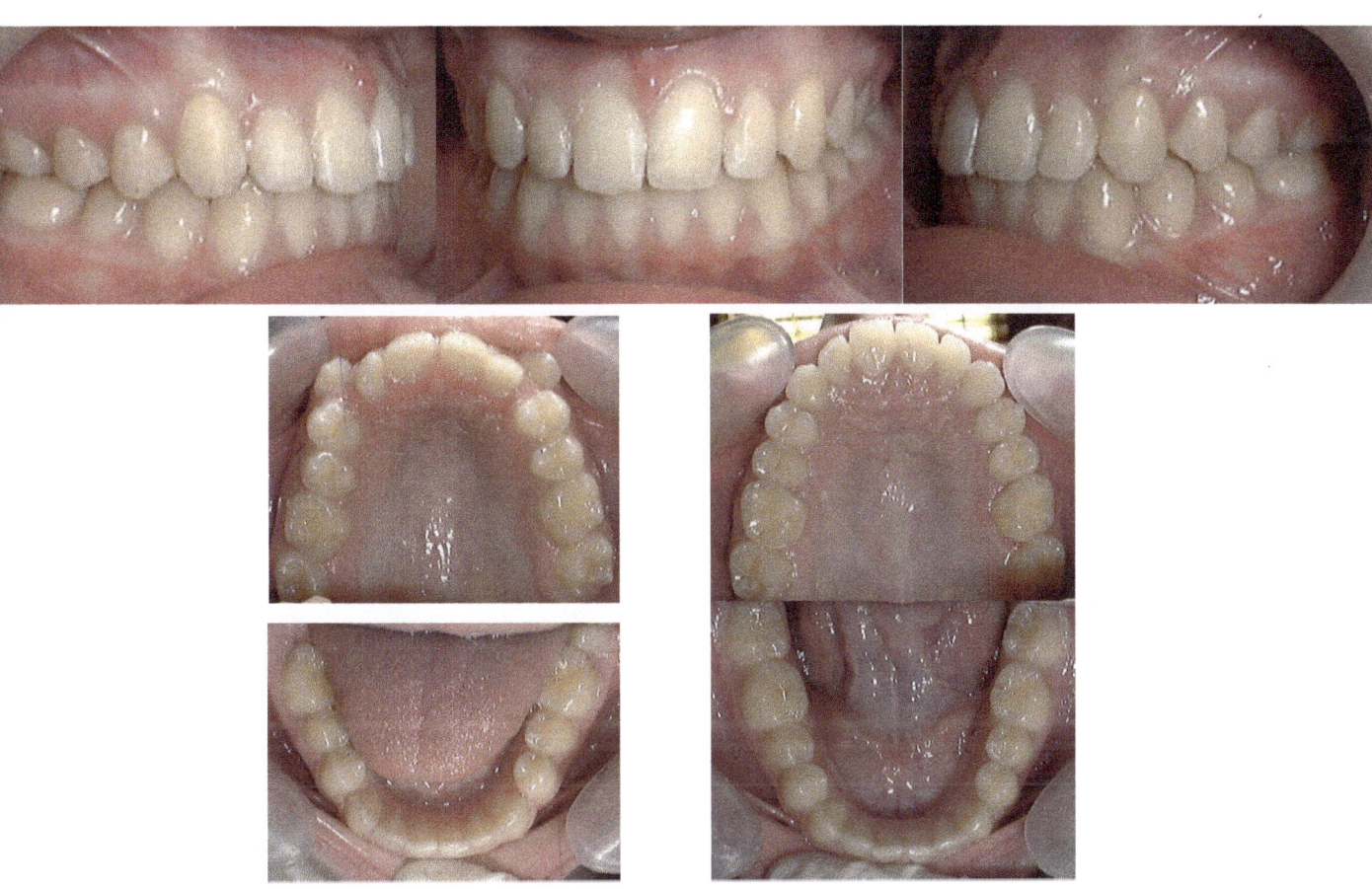

TransForce Orthodontics For A Brilliant Smile!

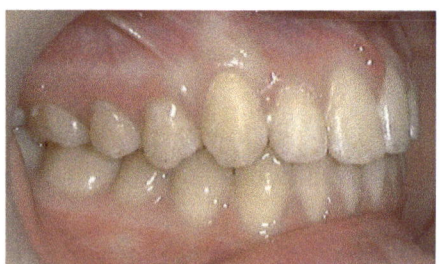 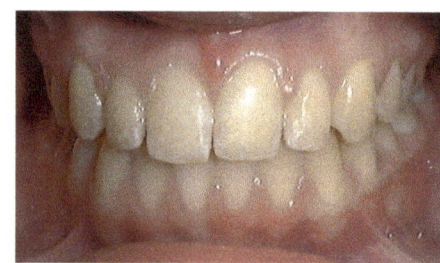 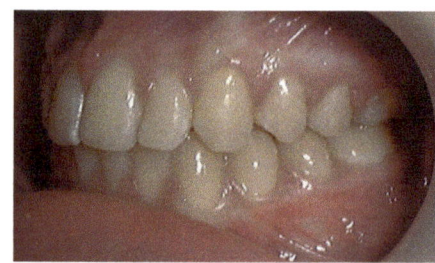

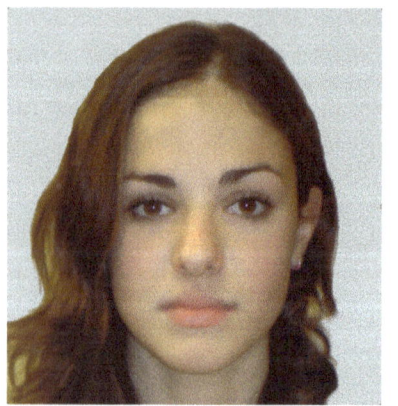 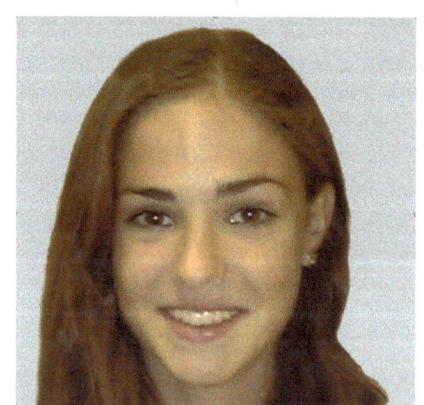 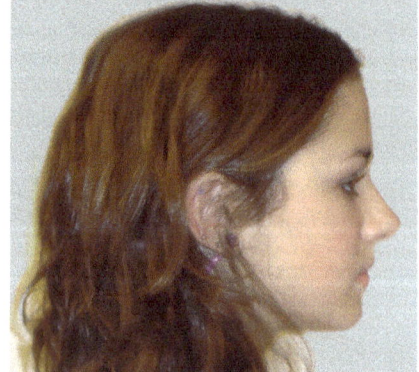

Two Years Later

Improved Facial Balance and a Beautiful Smile

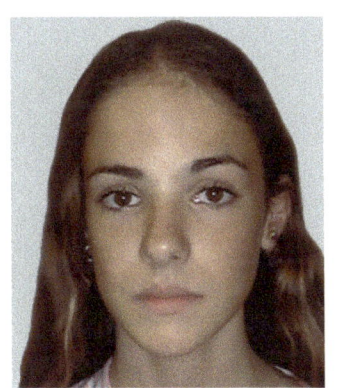 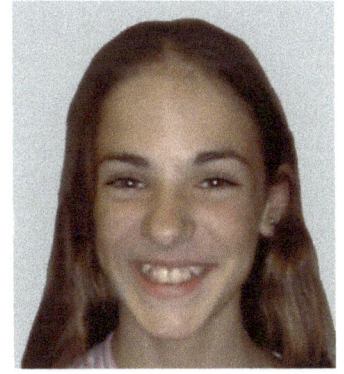 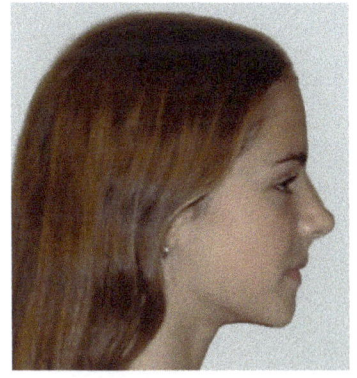

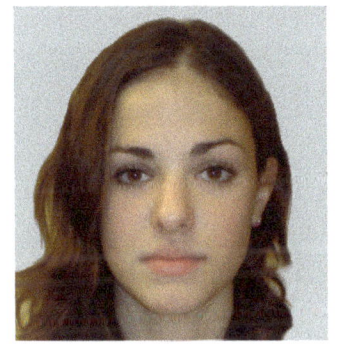 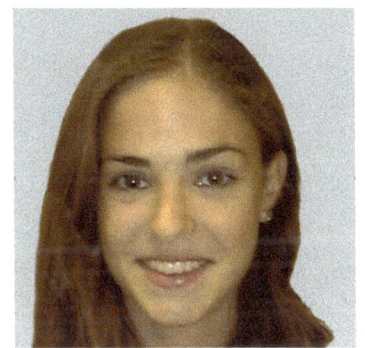 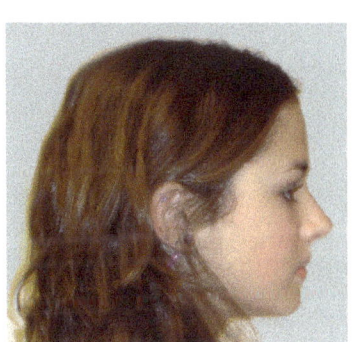

TransForce Treatment of Dental Asymmetry

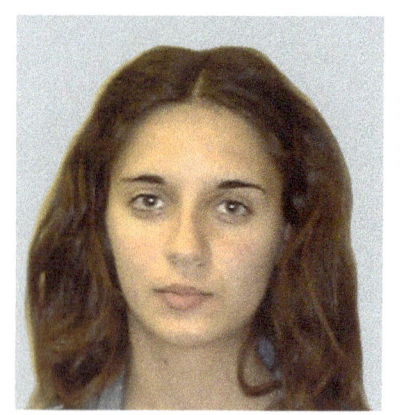 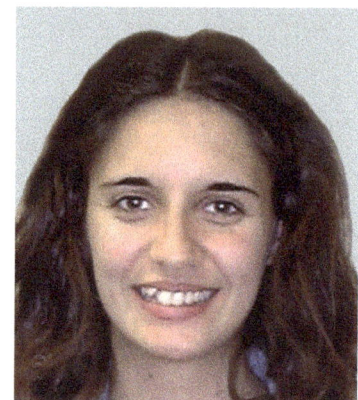 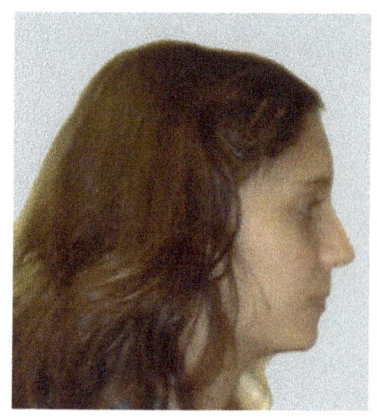

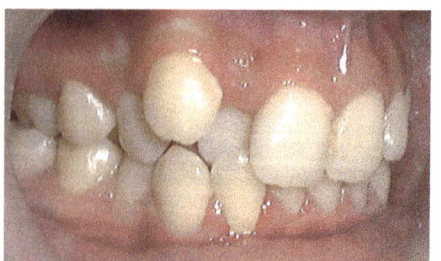 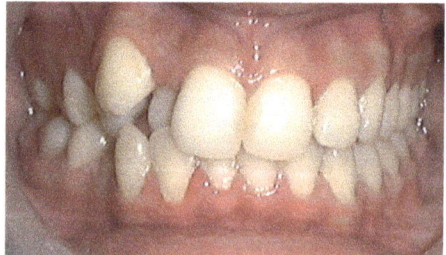 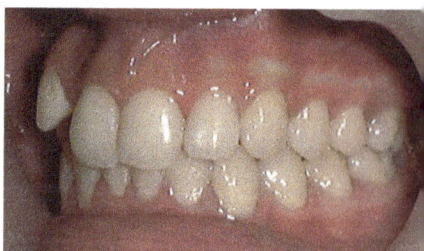

TransForce Palatal Expander

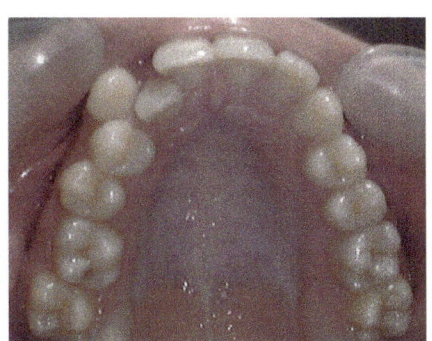 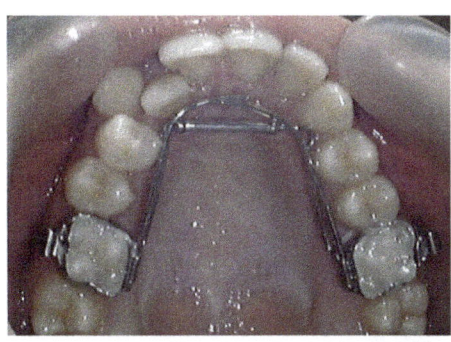 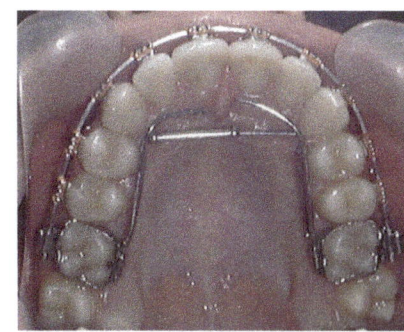

Lower Sagittal Corrects Asymmetry

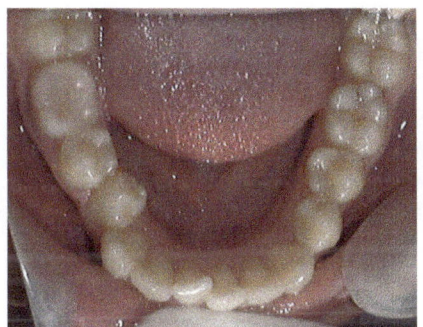 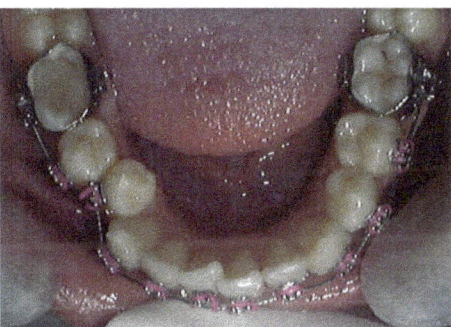 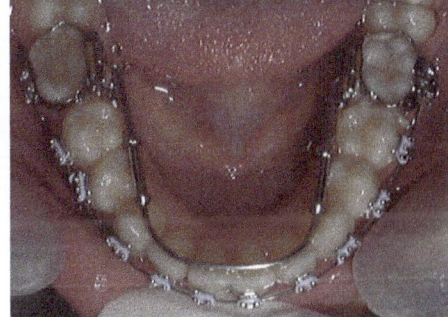

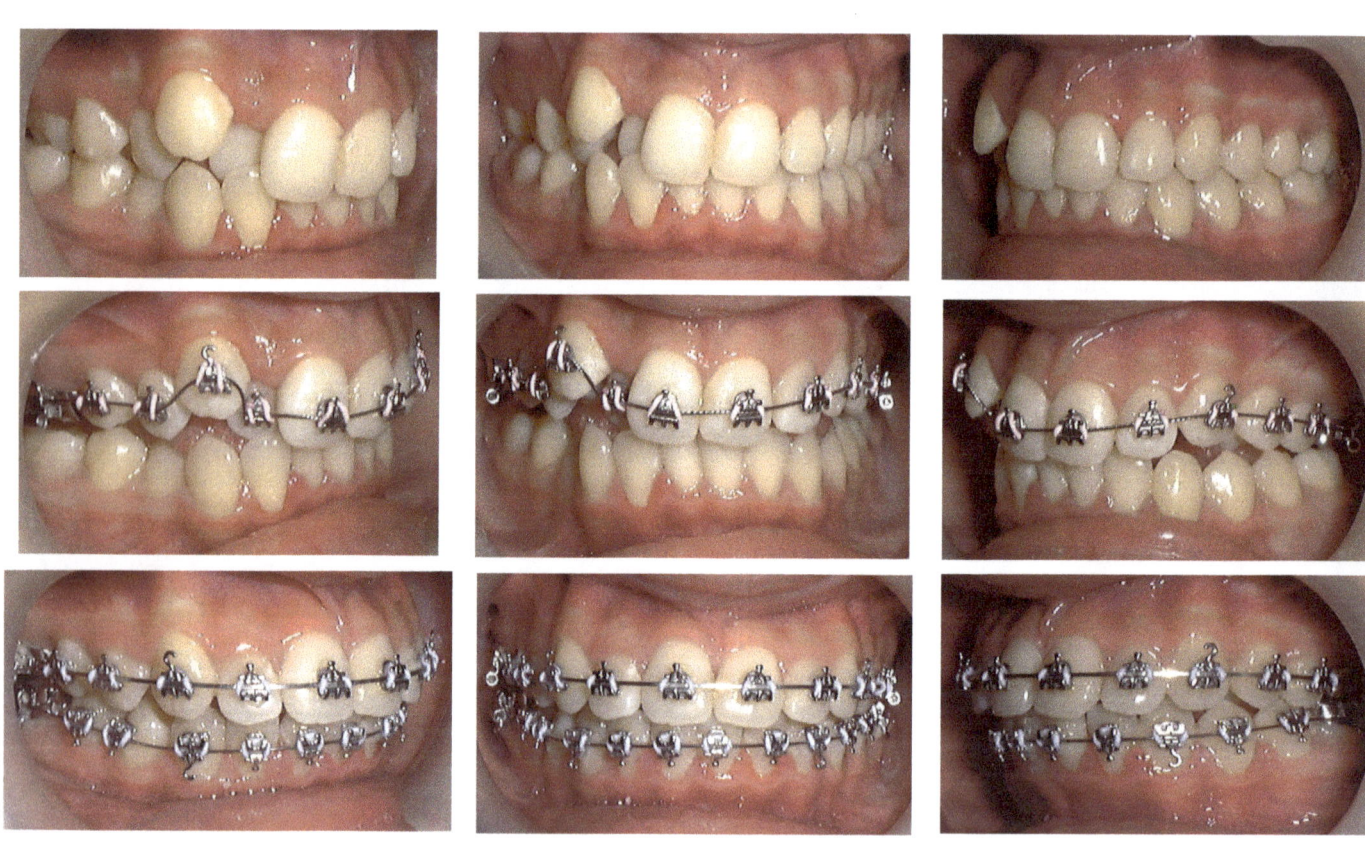

TransForce Palatal Expander

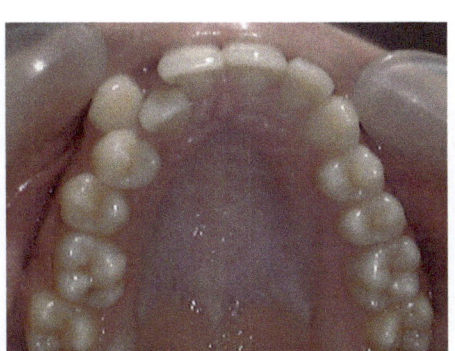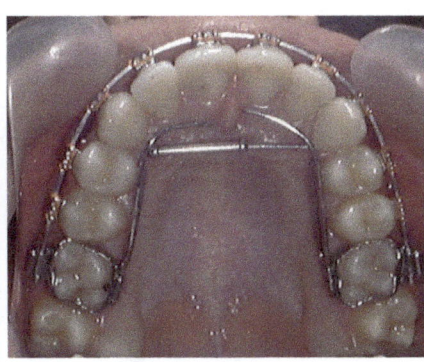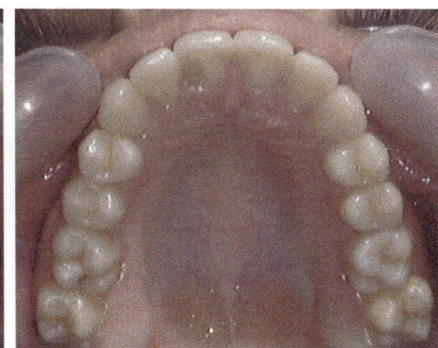

Lower Sagittal Corrects Asymmetry

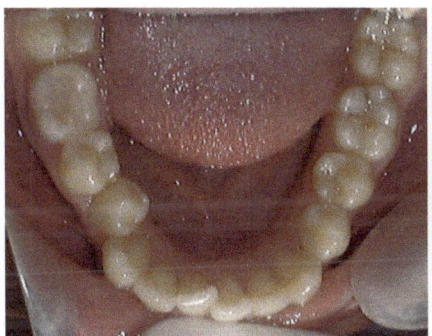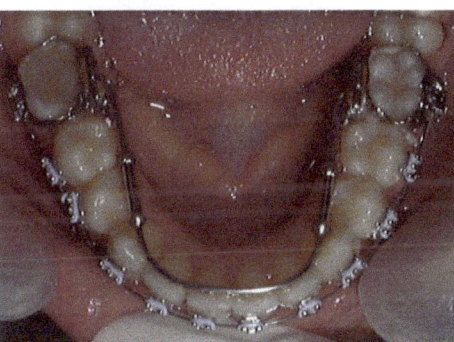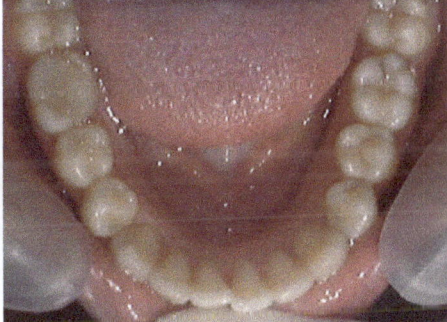

TransForce Palatal Expander

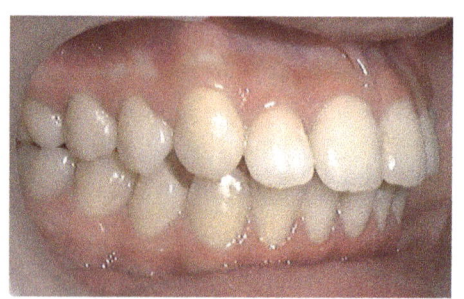 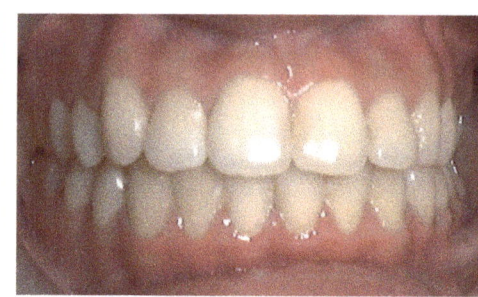 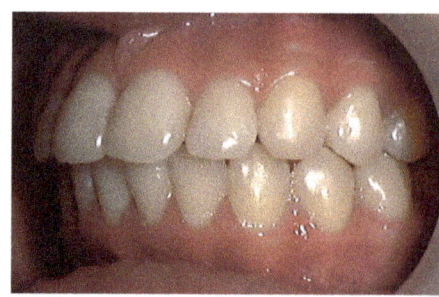

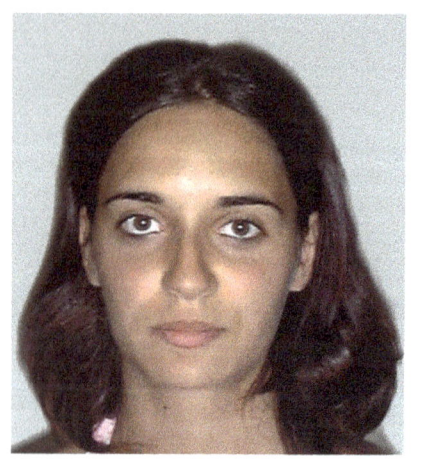 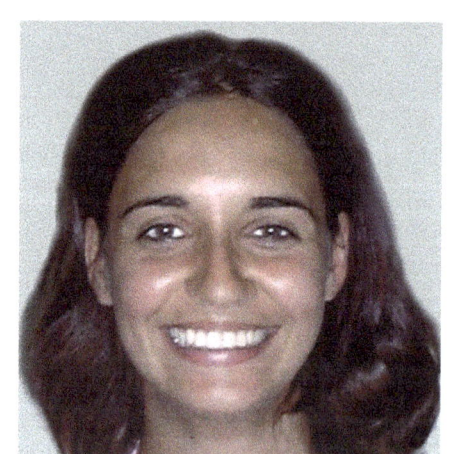 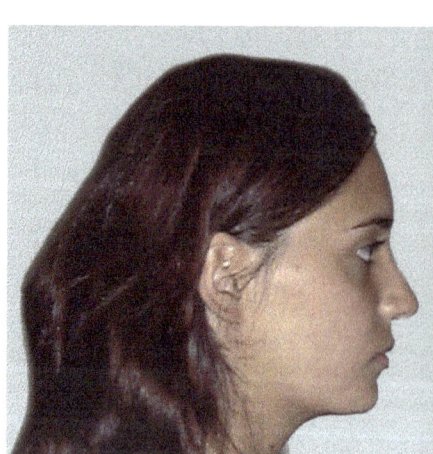

TransForce Treatment of Dental Asymmetry

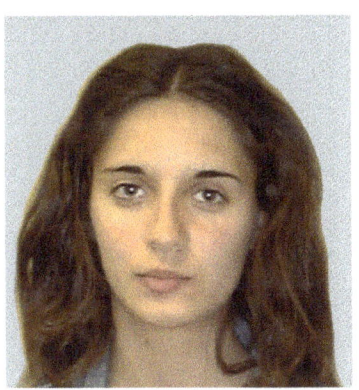 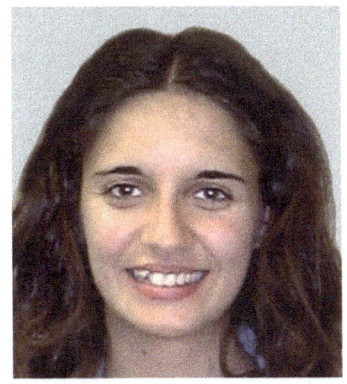 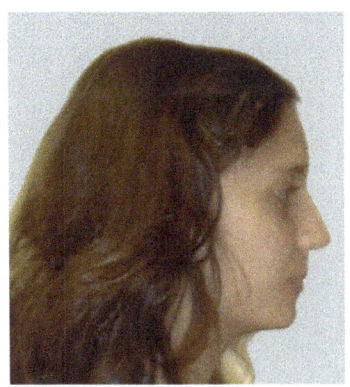

The Prize is a Brilliant Smile

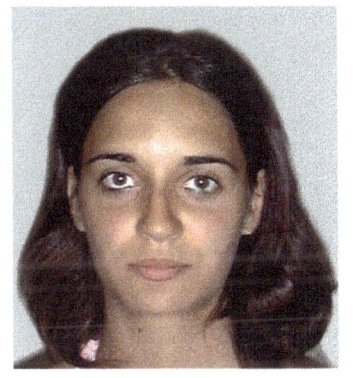 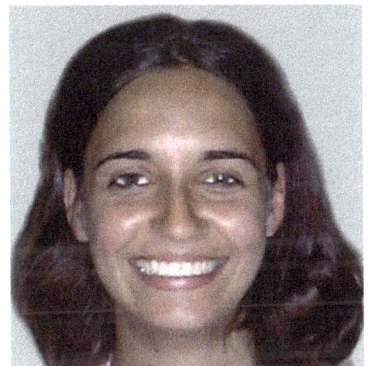 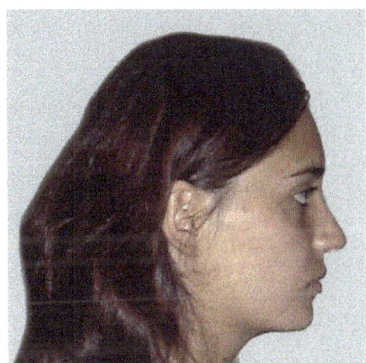

TransForce Orthodontics

- Non compliance - Fixed/Removable
- Sagittal and Transverse appliances
- Invisible upper & lower appliances
- Low continuous forces reduce discomfort & trauma
- Little or no adjustment required after fitting
- Reduce chair time by 50% !!!
- Integrates with labial & lingual brackets
- Integrates with Invisible Appliances
- Ideal for adult treatment

Try it - You'll like it !

New Horizons in Orthodontics

New Horizons in Orthodontics is a fundamental challenge to the orthodontic techniques of the present day. This account of contemporary orthodontic technique opened with a statement that the rate of technological change in contemporary society is accelerating and orthodontics is not exempt from this process. It is only human to be comfortable with familiar concepts and techniques and to resist progress. The danger of complacency applies equally in the academic or clinical environment.

In challenging the status quo the burden of proof rests with the innovator and understandably there is a time lag between the development of new techniques and their acceptance by academic and clinical representatives of the profession. I have been a passionate advocate of New Horizons in Orthodontics striving to keep pace with changes in technology and advancing knowledge of the specialty of orthodontics. I believe we are approaching a revolution in orthodontic technique, with rapid advances in digital technology and artificial intelligence. We should be aware of the effects of these changes on our specialty.

It is already evident that computer technology can usurp the role of the orthodontist. Already today treatment is planned by scanning the dentition and formulating a plan based on the teeth by computerised orthodontics. However this is a limited plan based only on moving the teeth. In my early days in orthodontics I realised that the definition of orthodontics does not take into account our role in the health and welfare of our patients, beyond the objective of straight teeth. It is no longer acceptable only to aim to correct the 'social six front teeth.

As specialists we must respect the importance of diagnosis and treatment planning not only in orthodontic terms, but also with attention to the wider aspect of airway and the impact of our techniques on the health of our patients.

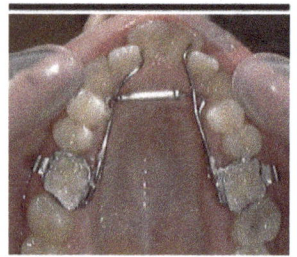

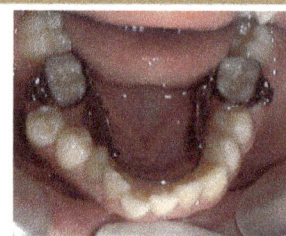

TransForce Orthodontics
Invisible TransForce Appliances

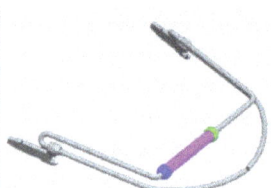

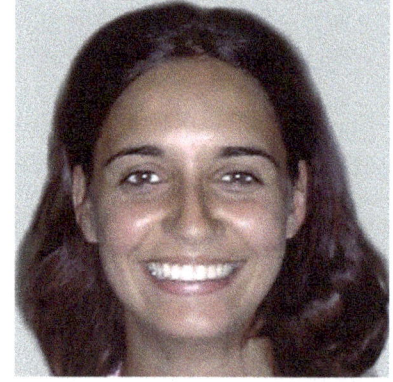

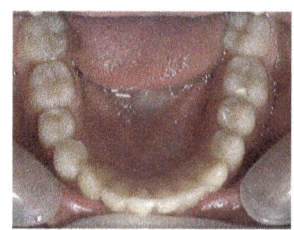

TransForm Your Orthodontics

William J Clark

B.D.S., D.D.O., D.D.Sc., F.D.S.R.C.S. Eng

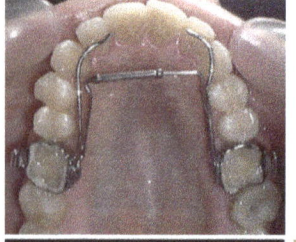